DIGIT RATIO

*A Pointer to Fertility,
Behavior, and Health*

John T. Manning

RUTGERS UNIVERSITY PRESS
New Brunswick, New Jersey, and London

Library of Congress Cataloging-in-Publication Data

Manning, John T., 1942–
    Digit ratio : a pointer to fertility, behavior, and health / John T. Manning.
        p. cm. — (The Rutgers series in human evolution)
    Includes bibliographical references and index.
    ISBN 0-8135-3029-6 (cloth: alk. paper) — ISBN 0-8135-3030-X (pbk. : alk. paper)
        1. Fingers—Sex differences.   2. Sex differentiation.   3. Sex differences.
    4. Embryology, Human.   I. Title.   II. Series.

    QM548 .M36 2002
    612.6—dc21   2001019836

British Cataloging-in-Publication information is available from the British Library.

Manufactured in the United States of America

To Olive, Linda, and Ruth

Contents

Figures

Tables

Preface and Acknowledgments

Evolutionary biologists are fascinated by the differences between males and females. Some of us are also enthusiastic about the potential for sexual selection theory to say something about human behavior and human illness. In pursuit of this many, including myself, have focused our work on sexually dimorphic traits which acquire their sex difference at puberty. This is a pragmatic decision because sexual differentiation is profoundly influenced by prenatal events. When we remember this, we pay lip service to the effects of testosterone, which acts on the fetus from as early as week eight of pregnancy. However, we then press on with our work regarding sexual dimorphisms in height and weight, breast size and asymmetry, waist:hip ratio, and jaw size. Of course we can learn much from sex differences that originate or are highly accentuated at puberty, but the reality is that we work on things that can be worked on. In utero effects are difficult if not impossible to measure, and behaviors and illnesses manifested in adults cannot be directly related to their prenatal etiology. Some colleagues, particularly those interested in the fetal origins of disease, have made inroads into these problems by looking at variables such as birth weight and expected birth weight. Much has been learnt in this way, but fetal conditions largely remain a mystery to us. The need is to identify a trait which is fixed in utero and which is sensitive to fetal concentrations of testosterone and estrogen. In this book I explore the hypothesis that the ratio of the length of the 2nd and 4th digit is such a trait.

The ratio between 2nd (the index finger) and 4th (the ring finger) digit length (2D:4D) tends to be lower in males compared to females. That is, men tend to have longer 4th digits compared to their 2nd than do women. Anatomists and anthropologists have known this for more than 100 years (Baker 1888; Phelps 1952). A similar curiosity, the distribution of hair on the dorsal surface of the fingers, has also been known for many years. Hair growth on the middle phalanx is more luxuriant on the 4th digit and least well developed on the 2nd digit, and this growth is dependent on testosterone (Winkler and Christiansen 1993). Taken together these apparently unconnected anecdotes may mean that prenatally a number of tissues which make up the 4th digit are sensitive to testosterone. There is evidence from fetal material that relative finger length is fixed by the end of week 14. Low 2D:4D ratios could correlate with high fetal testosterone and low fetal estrogen concentrations. The sex difference in the trait is not pubertal in origin, and common sense tells us it is not important in mate choice (although common sense is sometimes wrong). So it has not attracted much attention. However, it may be an indicator of steroid hormone levels at an important period for brain organization, sexual orientation, and the formation of the heart and major blood vessels and of the breasts.

Intriguingly there is much folklore associated with the 4th digit. It is known as the annulus or ring finger, because from Roman times it has been associated with the wearing of rings. Often a ring on this finger indicated the marital or reproductive status of the wearer. In some cultures the 4th digit is said to have a direct connection to the heart and to indicate the health of the heart by its length (Sorell 1968). Some anatomists and artists have regarded a long 4th digit relative to the 2nd as primitive and "simian like" and have pointed to its pronounced development in many nonhuman primates and in particular arboreal primates (Schultz 1924). Casanova claimed he was well endowed when it came to ring finger length relative to his index finger. He brought this, rather aggressively, to the attention of an artist friend who had a longer index finger than ring finger (Casanova's diaries 1997; quoted by Peters et al. 2000). In the arts and in palmistry, vague connections with creativity, musical ability, and an "atavistic or primitive" nature have all been ascribed to a long 4th digit (Sorell 1968).

These folklore associations may or may not be well founded in fact. I leave this to others to decide. This book is concerned with what science can tell us about the ratio. The topic is both old and new. It has been immensely interesting to read the old literature and to appreciate the careful work of the anatomists and anthropologists of the nineteenth and early twentieth centuries. The relationships of the 2D:4D ratio to prenatal steroidal hormones, sperm counts, fertility, disease, behaviors, and sports ability is a story of very recent work. It is my hope that this work will be taken forward in a rewarding program for research in the twenty-first century. The subject matter of the chapters is arranged in the following way:

In chapter 1 I discuss evidence that the 2D:4D ratio is sex-dependent. Interestingly it seems that the sex differences in the ratio are indeed real across geographical boundaries but also that between-population differences are probably much greater than between-sex differences. This is an important conclusion and we need to incorporate it into any discussion concerning 2D:4D ratios and population differences in disease predispositions and behaviors.

Chapter 2 reviews the evidence that low 2D:4D indicates high prenatal testosterone and sperm counts and that high 2D:4D is an indicator of high prenatal estrogen.

Chapter 3 concerns behaviors and traits, e.g., assertiveness, status, aggression, and attractiveness, which are important influences on reproductive success, while chapter 4 takes this further and discusses 2D:4D ratio as a predictor of lifetime reproductive success across cultures.

What of sex-dependent illnesses? Low 2D:4D and its association with the possibly neutral trait of handedness and with handicaps such as compromised verbal fluency, autism, and depression are in chapter 5. Chapter 6 is concerned with evidence that low 2D:4D is correlated with delays in development but that it may also indicate low probability of the important adult illnesses of coronary heart disease and breast cancer.

Chapter 7 is perhaps the least straightforward for it concerns the relationship between 2D:4D and male and female homosexuality. Patterns of 2D:4D ratio tend to support the position that homosexuality is associated with hypermasculinization in utero.

I have indulged my own interest in sexual selection in chapters 8 and 9. The former concerns music and 2D:4D ratio; the latter, sports, particularly football, and the ratio. Readers may find my sexual selection arguments provocative because they are applied to humans or because they concern activities which are not normally regarded as explicable in terms of sexual selection. Please remember it is the data in these chapters that are of primary importance. Interesting or provocative interpretations are often less durable than data. If the models are wrong, the data remain to be interpreted. Nevertheless, the patterns of 2D:4D ratios revealed in these data are consistent with the viewpoint that sexual selection shapes the behaviors of men and women in ways that echo its action on other species.

Finally, it is a great pleasure to acknowledge my colleagues who have helped in this endeavor. My work on the Jamaican Symmetry Project, led by Robert Trivers, came near the beginning of my interest in the 2D:4D ratio. Conversations with Bob and my close colleagues Randy Thornhill and Devendra Singh have always been a delight and have been important in shaping my ideas. This work has also led me outside my own discipline. Peter Bundred has helped immensely with the investigations on coronary heart disease, and his cardiac rehabilitation clinics were always places of great interest. Sam Leinster has been patient and helpful amid the stress of busy breast cancer clinics. Bernard Brabin and Loretta Brabin led me through the complexities of parasitic infections and their sexually dimorphic expression. Peter Pharoah provided an excellent opportunity to work on fetal growth. Chris Dowrick and Susan Martin gave authoritative background on depression. Simon Baron-Cohen and his group led me through the intricacies of autism. Geoff Sanders has helped with sex-dependent cognitive abilities. Marc Breedlove and Dennis McFadden with sexual orientation. Iwan Lewis-Jones, with his humor and tolerance, facilitated my work in fertility clinics. Rogan Taylor made it possible for me to meet football players with talents from the gods. Many more colleagues and students have collected data, and I offer my thanks to them all. It is wonderful to dip one's toes or, perhaps more appropriately, one's digits in other disciplines. These colleagues have made it possible. Of course any misconceptions or naivete associated with the work remain mine.

DIGIT RATIO

CHAPTER 1

Sex and Population Differences

At first sight the essence of the uterine environment appears to be protection. The fetus differentiates and grows, apparently isolated from the harsh Darwinian world experienced by children and adults. However, this impression of an idyll with its watery, membranous peace is misleading. It is essentially the result of inaccessibility. Common-sense observation can make little of prenatal differentiation and the scientist, bound about by ethical considerations, is often forced to make do with animal models. If there were ready access to prenatal development we would most likely see evidence for gene action which carries with it the familiar balance of advantage and disadvantage. Natural selection removes harmful genes from populations, but the power of selection is blunted when a gene has good and bad influences. This is likely to be true in the uterine environment, and variations in prenatal development may well underlie the variations in the behavior, fertility, and health of children and adults. The genes involved may give some individuals a bad start in life or predispose them to ill health or infertility in later life. In others they may confer robust physical and mental health and fertility. In order to understand the prenatal causes of ill health and why such genes are maintained in the population we require a "window" into uterine conditions. By necessity the window has to be a developmental record which has been fixed during prenatal life, preferably toward the end of the first trimester, when important organ systems are still being formed. My thesis in this book is that the relative lengths of the 2nd and 4th digits (2D:4D) provides a developmental window which speaks to us about sex-related behavior, fertility, and health. If this is so the ratio will be important in our understanding of patterns of fecundity, behavior, illness, and even differences between human populations.

But first (a) how are the 2nd and 4th digits measured; (b) how does the ratio differ between sexes and when in ontogeny does the difference arise; and (c) how does the 2D:4D ratio differ between species and human populations?

Measurement

Look at the hands in figure 1.1. Hand A is that of a man, and B is a woman's hand. The 2nd or index finger and the 4th or ring finger present an appearance of symmetry on either side of the long 3rd or middle

1

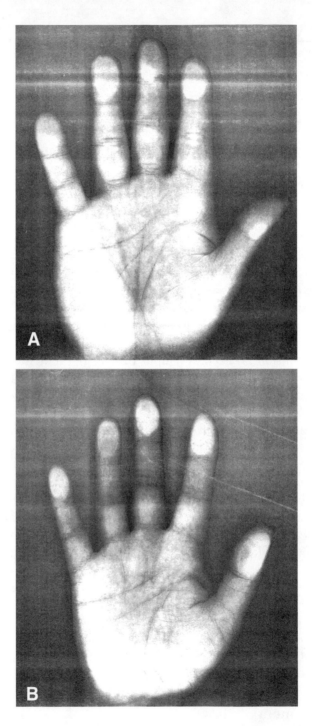

Figure 1.1. (A) The right hand of a Caucasian male with a 2D:4D ratio of 0.92. This is a low ratio for male Caucasians. (B) The right hand of a Caucasian female with a 2D:4D ratio of 1.00. This ratio is close to the mean in many female Caucasian samples.

finger. However, if one measures from the basal crease of the digits to the tip you will find that in the male hand the length of the index finger is 92% that of the ring finger. In other words, the ratio of 2nd:4th is 0.92. The female hand has a 2nd digit that is approximately the same length as the 4th digit. It's 2D:4D ratio is therefore 1.00.

Can the ratio be measured accurately? Consider data obtained from the 2nd and 4th digits of 300 hands from as many subjects. Each digit was measured twice using vernier calipers measuring to 0.01 mm. Using repeated measures ANOVA analysis we can compare the error mean squares (i.e., the differences between the repeated measurements) and the groups mean squares (i.e., the differences between the subjects). The ratio between the two (the F ratio) can then be tested to determine whether the differences between subjects are significantly larger than the errors in measurement. Considering the 2nd digit we find that $F = 341.81$ and $p = < 0.0001$. This means that differences between subjects are more than 340 times greater than measurement error. A similarly large F value was found for the 4th digit ($F = 375.75$, $p = < 0.0001$). However, we are concerned with the accuracy of measuring the 2D:4D ratio. In these data $F = 64.75$, $p = < 0.0001$ for 2D:4D. That is, differences in 2D:4D ratio between subjects are 65 times greater than its measurement error. A further indication of the accuracy of the measurement of the 2D:4D ratio is given by the intraclass correlation coefficient or repeatability (r_1) of the measurements. This is calculated as follows:

$$r_1 = \text{Groups MS} - \text{Error MS/(Groups MS} + \text{Error MS)}$$

For the 2nd digit $r_1 = 0.99$, for the 4th $r_1 = 0.99$, and for the 2D:4D ratio $r_1 = 0.97$. Therefore 2D:4D may be measured accurately.

Of course, measurement of digit length can be performed in a number of ways. For example, X-rays of hands may be used and measurements made from the proximal tip of the proximal phalanx (i.e., the finger bone which is closest to the palm) to the distal tip of the distal phalanx. Figure 1.2 shows the relationship between 2D:4D ratios calculated from measurements from X-rays and from soft tissue from 136 Jamaican children. The 2D:4D ratios correlate quite well. This is despite the fact that the soft-tissue measurements of the digits were taken from approximately halfway along the proximal phalanx whereas bone measurements began at the proximal end of the phalanx. In addition, the X-rays were taken 2.5 years before the photocopies. That there were significant relationships between the 2D:4D ratios from the two types of measurements also suggests that the ratio remains stable in children across periods of rapid growth.

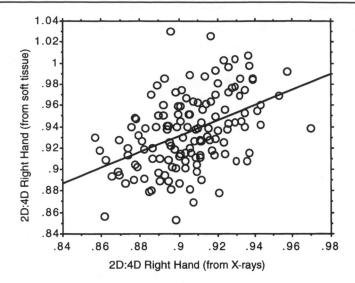

Figure 1.2. 2D:4D ratios calculated from hand X-rays and soft-tissue measurements made from photocopies of the hand in 136 Jamaican children. The photocopies were made 2.5 years after the X-rays. These two different methods of measurement made at different times in development produced similar results ($r = 0.45$, $F = 34.23$, $p = 0.0001$).

It is not usually practical to measure 2D:4D ratio from X-rays. In general in this book I refer to soft-tissue measurements taken directly from the hand using vernier calipers or made from photocopies of the palm of the hand or from "ink prints" of the ventral surface of the phalanges. Comparisons between 2D:4D ratios from the hand and from photocopies of the hand have shown the latter method to produce similar results. For example, the 2nd and 4th digits of 30 hands were measured from the hands and from photocopies of the hands. The 2D:4D ratios calculated from these two methods showed significant similarities ($r_1 = 0.88$, $F = 15.86$, $p = 0.0001$).

Sex Differences and Their Ontogeny

Many traits showing sex differences become obvious at puberty, e.g., height and weight differences; dimorphisms in jaw size and thickness of brow ridges; and hip, waist, and shoulder differences. Before puberty there may be little in the way of sex differences.

Puberty and Sex Differences

While breasts are thought to be typical of women, prenatal breast development is identical in males and females. The breast forms from the mid-thoracic persistence of the ectodermal mammary ridge, which initially extends on each side from the base of the forelimb to the hind limb (Sadler 1985). An area in the mid-thoracic region penetrates the underlying mesenchyme to give rise to the lactiferous ducts. The ducts empty into an epithelial pit from which the nipple forms. These changes are the same in males and females. In fact at birth 80% of both male and female babies produce milk. No further development occurs until puberty when estrogenic changes stimulate marked breast development in females. Approximately 38% of males may show early pubertal gynecomastia or breast enlargement as testicular estrogen increases before adult concentrations of testosterone reach maximum levels. However, pubertal gynecomastia resolves in 92% of boys by 16 years. The sexes are then markedly dimorphic in their breast development until the onset of senile gynecomastia in middle age when around 30% of men show breast enlargement, rising to 60% by the seventh decade (Gateley 1998).

Similar temporal patterns of sexual dimorphism may be seen in the skeleton and are detailed by Knight (1991). In the skull there are a number of features that become accentuated at puberty but are modified with age so that discriminant function analysis may best determine sex between approximately the twentieth to the fifty-fifth year. The male skull is more rugged and has greater development of muscle ridges than the female skull. Compared to females the male supraorbital ridge, mastoid process, palate, teeth, and mandible are larger. The male mandible has a squarer symphysis or chin region; the angle between the body and the ramus is more upright; the condyles and the ramus and the coronoid process are larger than those in females.

Prepubertal Sex Differences

Unlike the skull, sexual dimorphisms in the pelvis may be seen in weak form in children and even at the fetal stage. Males have a more rugged pelvis for muscle attachments with higher iliac blades and a narrower suprapubic angle. Many of the sex differences in the pelvis relate to childbirth. For example, the pelvic inlet is more circular in females, while that of the male is more heart-shaped as the result of the position of the sacrum. The sacrum is wider in females with a shallower curve, while the curve in the male is continuous and the coccyx may even project forward. After puberty the relatively wider pelvis in women leads to a difference in the angle that the shaft of the femur makes with the vertical. That is, the slope of the shafts is greater in women in order that the lower ends of the femur sit horizontally on the tibia.

Many of these differences are obvious to us because they are associated with sexual attraction and mate choice. It is no surprise that puberty modifies and increases these sexual dimorphisms. We are more interested in prenatal sexual differences, which may be very subtle but which could provide us with information on developmental conditions in utero. The arm may be rich in such traits. A perforated olecranon fossa at the lower end of the humerus is more common in females than males (female to male ratio of 3.7:1; Knight 1991). Interestingly, there is a difference in side in the sex-dependent expression of this trait. In females a perforated olecranon fossa is more frequent on the left than the right. The asymmetry of elbow thickness (left elbow–right elbow) may also show sex differences. Trivers et al. (1999) have reported higher elbow asymmetry in female Jamaican children compared to males. The asymmetry was strongly directional, with left elbows thicker than right in both sexes. Continuing down the arm the length of the forearm relative to the humerus or to the height of the individual is greater in men than in women (Tanner 1990; Knight 1991). However, it is in the digits and in particular the 2D:4D ratio where our greatest opportunity may lie to view a proxy for prenatal concentrations of sex steroids. Why is this so?

The overall pattern of development in multicellular animals is controlled by Homeobox or *Hox* genes. In humans there are 39 *Hox* genes arranged in four clusters designated *Hoxa* to *Hoxd* (Scott 1997). Two groups of genes *Hoxa* and *Hoxd* control both the development of the testes and ovaries and also (remarkably) the fingers and the toes (Mortlock et al. 1996; Kondo et al. 1997). In humans mutations of *Hoxa,* in particular *Hoxa13,* may result in the hand-foot-genital syndrome, in which there are defects in the digits and urinogenital system (Mortlock and Innis 1997). In the limbs these include short first metacarpals, thumbs with reduced distal phalanges, abnormalities of the 2nd and 5th digits, fusion of the wrist bones, and short great toes resulting from a reduced first metatarsal and the distal phalanx. In the urinogenital system there may be a partially or completely divided uterus and a displaced urethral opening. Similarly, work with mice suggests that deregulation of *Hoxd* expression alters digit length and also causes genital malformations (Peichel et al. 1997; Herault et al. 1997). In humans *Hoxd* mutations may cause the condition synpolydactyly, which involves syndactyly of the 3rd and 4th digits, with digit duplication in the syndactylous web. Hand involvement is frequently asymmetrical, and mildly affected individuals may merely have short 4th digits. Males may also have genital malformations. Therefore, the ontogeny of the digits and that of the testes and ovaries share causal factors, and disruptions of one may be associated with disruptions of the other. Some of these disruptions are known to affect the development of the 2nd and 4th digits and the urinogenital system.

2D:4D and Sex Differences

If we are interested in the relationship between uterine conditions and sex-dependent behaviors and diseases, why is the 2D:4D ratio, rather than other aspects of the digits, a likely place to start? It has been known for more than 100 years that Caucasian men tend to have 4th digits longer than their 2nd digits, while Caucasian women tend to have 2nd longer than 4th (see Baker 1888; George 1930). Michael Peters, Kevin Mackenzie, and Pam Bryden (2002) have provided a fascinating and scholarly overview of the historical literature relating to 2D:4D. They show that the relative length of the 2nd and 4th digits has been variously calculated from measurements of the distal extent of the fingertips using the 3rd digit as standard, or by measuring absolute finger length from the basal crease of the finger, the skin fold in the gap between the fingers, or from the metacarpo-phalangeal joint. Many of the historical studies have found within-population sex differences in Caucasians, in that males tend to have lower values of 2D:4D ratios than females (Ecker 1875; Gruning 1886; George 1930; Phelps 1952). An inspection of the right-hand 2D:4D ratio from a sample of 1,052 Liverpool subjects (521 males and 531 females; see figure 1.3) shows that it has a more-or-less bell-shaped distribution and is lower in men than women, but with a very substantial overlap (Manning et al. 1998).

Of course, there are sex differences in body size, but the 2D:4D ratio is not strongly related to height in adults. For example, a sample of 100 Caucasian males and 100 Caucasian females with a mean age of 42.63 ± 8.80 years showed significant sex differences in right-hand 2D:4D (male mean 0.98 ± 0.04, female mean 0.99 ± 0.03, $t = 3.68$, $p = 0.0003$), and height (male mean 176.48 ± 6.80 cms, female mean 167.75 ± 5.78 cms, $t = 9.78$, $p = 0.0001$). However, 2D:4D was not significantly associated with height in men ($b = -19.58$, $F = 1.12$, $p = 0.29$) or in women ($b = -26.94$, $F = 1.23$, $p = 0.13$).

Do the sex differences in 2D:4D reside in the relative lengths of the digits themselves or in sex-dependent differences in the bones of the palm? The hand is made up of three segments—the wrist or carpus, the palm or metacarpus, and the fingers or phalanges (Gray 1858). The metacarpal bones, which are found in the palm, are five in number and each articulates proximally with the wrist and distally with the proximal bone or phalanx of a finger. The bones of the fingers are the phalanges; they number 14, 3 for each finger and 2 for the thumb. In the palm the metacarpal bone of the index finger is longer than the metacarpal of the ring finger. Interestingly, in common with the metacarpals of the middle and little finger, the index metacarpal has attachments for five muscles but

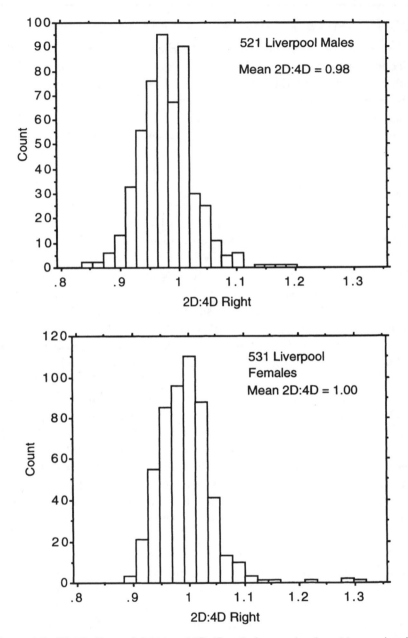

Figure 1.3. Distributions of right-hand 2D:4D ratio in samples from Liverpool males (n = 521) and females (n = 531). On average males have lower 2D:4D ratios than females (male mean 0.98 ± 0.03SD, female mean 1.00 ± 0.03SD, t = 3.31, p = 0.001). However, note the substantial overlap of the sexes in this U.K. sample.

the ring finger metacarpal has attachments for only three. In addition the phalanges of the index finger have attachments for seven muscles while the phalanges of the ring finger have six attachments. This may explain why the range of movement of the ring finger is less than for the index and other fingers. Wood-Jones (1941) has argued that 2D:4D ratio is independent of the ratio between the index metacarpal and the ring metacarpal. Phelps (1952) analyzed data from Pfitzner (1892) and found that the ratio between index and ring finger lengths was not correlated with the ratio between index and ring metacarpal lengths in males ($r = -0.12$) or females ($r = -0.01$). This supports the position that the 2D:4D ratio does not arise from metacarpal length but is an independent characteristic of the digits.

However, there is some evidence that the 2D:4D ratio is related to other sex-dependent features of the forearm. The length of the forearm (measured from the wrist) corrected for height tends to be greater in men than women (Tanner 1990). In a study of forearm length and 2D:4D ratio in 72 Liverpool men, Manning (manuscript) found that participants with long forearms relative to their height (right forearm length/height of the individual) had lower 2D:4D, i.e., a more "malelike ratio" than men with short forearms relative to their height who had a more "femalelike ratio." The negative relationship between forearm length and 2D:4D ratio was significant ($r = -0.30, p = 0.0009$). It is not known whether other features of the arm correlate with 2D:4D ratio. Peters et al. (2000) did not find a relationship between 2D:4D and either hand length or hand width in a Canadian sample of 71 males and 251 females. However, hand length and width can also be measured from dermatoglyphic markers that are determined prenatally.

The 2D:4D ratio may correlate with patterns of dermatoglyphic ridges. The fingertips have ridges that are fixed in number by the fourth month of fetal life, and most individuals have a higher ridge count on their right hand (Holt 1968). There are sex differences in this pattern. The total ridge count is higher in males than in females (Penrose 1967), and the incidence of a higher left count is greater in women than in men (Holt 1968; Kimura and Carson 1995). Hand width and length may also be measured using dermatoglyphic markers at the base of the 2nd and 5th digits and near the wrist crease. The combination of early determination and marked sexual dimorphism suggests that 2D:4D and dermatoglyphic pattern may be correlated.

Manning, Stevenson, Bundred, and Pharoah (manuscript) have considered the relationships between dermatoglyphics and 2D:4D in a sample of very low birth weight children. This was a cohort study of 206 children who had a birth weight of less than or equal to 1,500 g. Ink prints of the children's hands were taken at age 15 years. Finger length and dermatoglyphics were measured from the ink prints. The basal crease of the digits was not apparent in most prints. Measurements were therefore made from the proximal crease of the middle phalanx to the tip of the finger. The proximal crease was sufficiently well defined to make possible the calculation of 2D:4D ratio in 126 right and 143 left hands. In order to classify the pattern of dermal ridges on the fingertips it is necessary to count the triradii. A triradius is a meeting place of three ridges that form an angle of about 120°. There are three basic types of fingerprint patterns: loops, whorls, and arches. The defining characteristic of a loop is that the direction of a parallel group of lines turns through two right angles. When two loops are fused into a circle, the pattern is a whorl. If the lines are curved but without true pattern, they form an arch. Loops and whorls have two triradii; arches have none. The ridge counts are made from the triradius to the center of the pattern. Therefore, loops and whorls have two ridge counts each, but arches have none (Penrose 1967). Triradii can also be used to indicate the form of the hand. There is usually a triradius on the palm at the base of each finger and at the base of the palm near to the wrist crease. Lines drawn from the palmar triradius to the 2nd and 5th digit triradii mark an angle (ATD) that is related to hand morphology. A short, broad hand has a large ATD; a long, narrow hand a small ATD. The relationships between 2D:4D and ridge counts on the 2nd and 4th digits were examined. All associations were negative; i.e., low values of 2D:4D were related to high ridge counts. The association between 2D:4D and the 4th digit of the right hand was significant ($p = 0.002$; see figure 1.4). There were also negative relationships between 2D:4D and ATD. Low values of 2D:4D were associated with a short, broad hand, i.e., high ATD. The relationship was significant for the left hand (right $b = -24.26$, $F = 2.43$, $p = 0.12$; left $b = -31.19$, $F = 5.73$, $p = 0.02$). In all there are six relationships reported here. Correction for multiple tests leaves the association between 2D:4D and 4th digit ridge counts significant ($p = 0.002$ corrected to $p = 0.006$). These data suggest that low values of 2D:4D ratio are related to high dermatoglyphic ridge counts and a short, broad hand. In addition, because patterns of dermatoglyphics are fixed in utero, the findings strongly support an early origin of the 2D:4D ratio. However, the measurements are from a sample of subjects (very low birth weight children) who may have experienced high prenatal stress. We must be cautious in assuming these associations apply to most individuals.

The question of the sex-dependent inheritance of the 2D:4D ratio has been addressed by Phelps (1952). For simplicity she suggested a model

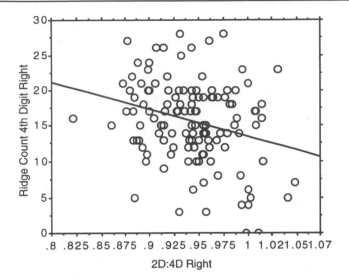

Figure 1.4. The relationship between 2D:4D of the right hand and dermatoglyphic ridge count on the 4th digit of the right hand in 126 very low birth weight children. The equation for the line is $y = -38.201x + 51.641$.

with three phenotypes for relative digit length: (a) 2D < 4D, (b) 2D = 4D, and (c) 2D > 4D. In a Caucasian sample of the left hands of students and staff from the University of Texas, it was found that 2D < 4D was most frequent among males (59%) and 2D > 4D most frequent (57%) among females. These sex-dependent differences in frequencies were similar to those found in a Caucasian sample from Canada (2D < 4D = 65% in males and 2D > 4D = 47% in females; George 1930). In order to explain the sex-dependent phenotypic expression of 2D:4D ratio, Phelps suggested a genetic model, which she adapted from a suggestion used to explain the genetic control of frontal baldness. Letting the allele for a relatively short 2nd digit be I^s and a relatively long 2nd digit be I^l, there are then three possible genotypes (I^sI^s, I^sI^l, and I^lI^l). Phelps found that data from familial analyses were consistent with heterozygotes (I^sI^l) having a relatively short 2nd digit in males but a relatively long 2nd digit in females. If this is so, then 2D < 4D would be more common in males than females. This is not the whole picture, however, because the lowest values of 2D:4D ratios are found in males and the highest in females. In order to explain this it was suggested that modifiers on the X chromosome were responsible for the sex-related differences in continuous variation seen in the ratio. Phelps's model is valuable as a first attempt to show sex-influenced genetic control of 2D:4D. However, the three phenotypes of 2D < 4D, 2D = 4D, and

2D > 4D are not always common in many populations. For example, Finns, South Africans, and Jamaicans have few individuals with a 2D > 4D phenotype. It is more likely that 2D:4D is under polygenic control. Interestingly, the sexually dimorphic pattern in the 2D:4D ratio may also be seen in a weaker form in the ratio between the 2nd and the 3rd digit (2D:3D). Phelps (1952) found evidence for 2D:3D ratios to be lower in men than women. This may mean that the growth of the 3rd and 4th digits are under the control of the same factors.

Ramesh and Murty (1977) have also addressed the question of variation and inheritance of the 2D:4D ratio. Their sample was from a Reddy community of the Nalgonda District of India. Ramesh and Murty did not favor a simple Mendelian model of one locus segregating for two alleles. They rightly point out that 2D:4D is a continuously varying trait and calculate a heritability of 40 to 70% from parent-offspring regressions and full-sibling correlations within 190 families. Surprisingly, they found no evidence for sex differences in 2D:4D phenotypes or for the influence of sex-linked additive genes.

Support for a genetic influence on the 2D:4D ratio comes from data from the Jamaican Symmetry Project on 88 mother-child pairs. There was a significant positive relationship between the mean 2D:4D ratio of mothers and children ($r = 0.34$, $F = 11.34$, $p = 0.001$; see figure 1.5). There were also positive correlations between mean 2D:4D of mothers and their male and female children. The male relationship was significant and the female association close to significance (male children, $n = 43$, $r = 0.43$, $F = 9.70$, $p = 0.003$, Bonferroni corrected $p = 0.006$; female children, $n = 45$, $r = 0.27$, $F = 3.40$, $p = 0.07$). It is probably not appropriate to calculate heritability scores from these data because we have some evidence of assortative mating for 2D:4D. The associations may of course be inflated by a maternal effect. Marshall (2000) has presented evidence for heritability of 2D:4D in 41 father-child pairs and 64 mother-child pairs recruited from Caucasians resident in the Liverpool area. The samples showed no evidence of assortative pairing for 2D:4D. He found a significant positive association in father-child pairs that gave a heritability of 0.53 $\pm$ 0.17SE ($t = 3.88$, $p = 0.001$). The heritability for mother-daughter pairs was lower ($h^2 = 0.34 \pm 0.15$) but nevertheless significant ($t = 2.22$, $p = 0.03$). The mid-parent:offspring sample was small ($n = 27$) and gave a heritability of 0.32 $\pm$ 0.44, but this relationship was not significant ($t = 1.77$, $p = 0.09$). Together with the work of Ramesh and Murty (1977) these findings suggest there is a moderate level of heritability of 2D:4D. In chapter 5 I discuss a study of families that include children with autism. There was no evidence of assortative pairing for 2D:4D in these families, and mid-parent:offspring regression gave a heritability of 0.58 $\pm$ 0.19.

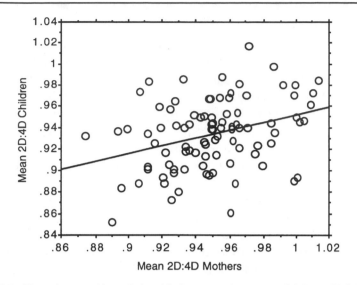

Figure 1.5. There is a positive relationship between the mean of right and left 2D:4D ratios of mothers and their children (subjects 88 Jamaican women and their children, $r = 0.34$, $p = 0.001$). This suggests that genes may well influence the formation of the 2D:4D ratio. However, on this evidence we cannot exclude the possibility of strong maternal effects.

When Is 2D:4D Established?

Regarding the ontogeny of the 2D:4D ratio, Phelps (1952) found that the full range of ratios, i.e., 2D:4D < 1, 2D:4D = 1, and 2D:4D > 1, was present in fetal material after the seventh week of pregnancy. In addition evidence that the 2D:4D ratios of parents were correlated with and similar to the 2D:4D ratios of their children led her to suggest that the ratios were fixed prenatally. Measurements of 56 human embryos and fetuses by Garn et al. (1975) provided further evidence of prenatal attainment of adult phalangeal ratios. They found that in the eighth and ninth intrauterine week there was a period of phalangeal elongation and that the tenth through thirteenth weeks are critical to a phalangeal reduction relative to the metacarpals. Relative proportions among phalangeal elements were closely similar to adult norms by the thirteenth or fourteenth week of pregnancy. This was a cross-sectional rather than a longitudinal study. The authors concluded that relative phalangeal proportions are established in the mesenchymal and cartilaginous hand models well before bone-collar and distal-tuft calcification. Support for an early origin of the sexually dimorphic nature of the ratio also comes from the work of Manning et al. (1998). They measured the 2nd and 4th digits of the right and left hands of 800 Merseyside subjects (400 males and 400 females). The age of the subjects ranged from 2 to 25 years. In the sample from 2 to 18 years, the participants consisted of 40 subjects (20 males and 20 females) for each year group, i.e., 40 participants aged 2 years, 40 aged 3 years, and so forth. The sample from 19 to 25 years consisted of 120 participants (60 males and 60 females). There were no obvious changes in 2D:4D ratio with age, and sexual dimorphism was present from an early age (see figure 1.6).

The Liverpool study showed little evidence for a change in 2D:4D at puberty. This question is further illuminated by considering mother-daughter pairs in relationship to 2D:4D and to waist:hip ratio (WHR). The length of the 2nd and 4th digits of the left and right hands together with the circumference of the waist and hips were measured in a sample of 34 Caucasian mother-daughter pairs from Liverpool (mothers' ages ranged from 27 to 51 years with a mean of 34.22 ± 7.31, and daughters' ages ranged from 7 to 9 years with a mean of 7.84 ± 0.85). The 2D:4D ratio of right and left hands were very similar, and an average of the right and left 2D:4D was calculated. Mothers had slightly higher 2D:4D ratio (mean 0.95 ± 0.03) than daughters (0.94 ± 0.03). However, subtracting the 2D:4D ratio of mothers from that of their daughters gave an average difference that was very close to zero (-0.007 ± 0.04) and that did not significantly differ from zero (one-sample t test, $t = 0.89$, $p = 0.38$). Contrast this with the WHR measurements. At puberty women tend to lay down fat on their hips but not on their stomach (Garn 1957). The ratio of the circumference of waist to hips therefore reduces. In this sample the mean WHR was lower for mothers (0.77 ± 0.07) than for daughters (0.83 ± 0.05). Subtracting the WHR of mothers from that of daughters resulted in a positive difference; i.e., on average mothers had lower WHR than daughters (mean 0.05 ± 0.08), and this difference was significantly higher than zero (one-sample t test, $t = 3.36$, $p = 0.002$). It should be noted that there is little in the way of sex differences in WHR before puberty. Data from the Jamaican Symmetry Project of measurements from children between 5 and 12 years of age show a mean WHR of 0.83 ± 0.05 for 140 boys and 0.84 ± 0.05 for 117 girls. The difference was not significant ($t = 1.71$, $p = 0.09$). It appears from these data that 2D:4D ratio changes very little at puberty in females. This is in strong contrast to the WHR of females, which shows a marked reduction at puberty.

A long-term longitudinal study is necessary to definitively establish whether 2D:4D changes during childhood, at puberty, and in middle or old age. However, the available evidence suggests that there are sex differences in 2D:4D at birth and that much of the between-individual differences in 2D:4D are established before birth. In this the 2D:4D ratio is very different from most other sexually dimorphic traits in humans.

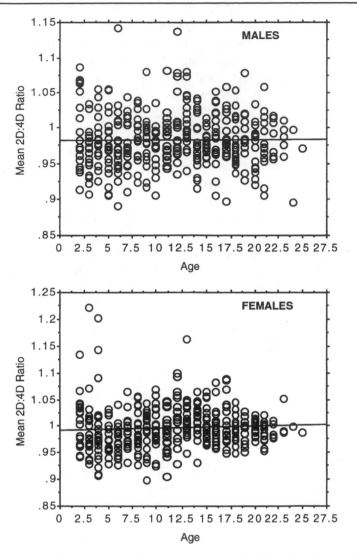

Figure 1.6. There is no evidence for a change in the 2D:4D ratio with age in 800 Merseyside males and females (400 males and 400 females) aged from 2 years to 25 years (males $r = 0.02$, $F = 0.09$, $p = 0.76$; females $r = 0.06$, $F = 1.25$, $p = 0.27$). Note there is no marked change in 2D:4D at puberty. This is an unusual feature in a sexually dimorphic trait.

A Function for the 4th Digit?

Thus far I have discussed 2D:4D without reference to the possible selective consequences of the different ratios. Peters et al. (2000) have speculated that differences in the distal length of the 2nd and 4th fingers may reduce the force and accuracy of throwing. They suggest that the 3rd digit is of central importance to the throw while the index and ring finger support and stabilize the middle finger. This interesting idea, which places the "throwing ape" at the center of our evolution, implies that selection will operate to ensure that the distal extent of the index and ring fingers will be equal. That they are not equal in most people may be because (a) the selective pressures favoring 2D:4D ratios of unity are weak or (b) there are other, more important reasons, for unequal lengths of the 2nd and 4th digit. One possibility is that the 2D:4D ratio, or at least the length of one of the digits relative to the hand as a whole, may be a display trait used in courtship. This appears to be unlikely at first sight given that the ratio seems to show little change at puberty. However, the 4th digit and its metacarpal have fewer muscle attachments and a reduced range of movement compared to that of the other digits, and may be less important in maintaining dexterity. The length of the ring finger, relative to that of the other digits, could tell us more about fertility status than about the dexterity of the hand. The 4th digit as a correlate of attractiveness is considered in chapter 3.

2D:4D Differences between Populations and between Species

The theme of this book is that 2D:4D ratio is an important correlate of a substantial suite of traits that are influenced by prenatal exposure to steroidal hormones. Are these relationships ancient so that they reach beyond human, primate, and even mammalian groups?

2D:4D and the Early Evolution of Hox Gene Control

If the sexual dimorphism in 2D:4D is related to the action of *Hox* genes, it may be that 2D:4D ratios show sex differences in many different species. *Hox* genes are highly conserved and show marked similarities across disparate taxa (Kondo et al. 1997). The common control of the formation of the urinogenital system and the extremities such as the fingers, the toes, and the penis may have originated in vertebrates during the transition from an aquatic to a terrestrial environment. This transition would tend to link the evolution of the pentadactyl or five-digit limb to that of the penis and a urinogenital system that facilitates fertilization and the successful early development of the young in a terrestrial environment. That is, a truly terrestrial animal requires efficient limbs for movement and an intromittent organ to ensure internal fertilization so that both locomotion and reproduction are possible on land (Kondo et al. 1997). In addition to changes in locomotion and reproduction the transition to land involves changes in the ears and the eyes. Parsimony in the genetic control of terrestrial adaptations may mean that 2D:4D could be correlated with sexually dimorphic traits in this limb/reproductive system/sensory organ complex of terrestrial traits.

The change from life in the water to life on land began some 400 million years ago in the lower Devonian with the primitive lobe-finned fish the Panderichthyids. These fish were predators found in shallow water, and they had lungs that would have allowed them to survive in oxygen-depleted water. Their eyes were positioned on top of the head and may have functioned above the water line. The evolutionary changes that followed are consistent with adaptation to a shallow-water, unpredictable habitat and have led to a suite of traits that were preadaptations for a terrestrial life. The changes included the acquisition of limbs, an excretory system that could cope with a shortage of water, and a reproductive system that ensured internal fertilization and early development independent of external water. These changes led to amphibians such as *Ichthyostega, Acanthostega,* and *Tulerpeton* in the upper Devonian and were completed by the true land vertebrates, the reptiles, which appeared 338 million years ago in the Carboniferous (Romer 1966; Zimmer 1998). Unlike the lobe-finned fish, the early amphibia had well-developed limbs. *Ichthyostega* had particularly powerful forelimbs, but *Acanthostega* had well-developed hind limbs and poorly differentiated forelimbs. Toes may have evolved to aid manipulation of thick waterside vegetation. The number of toes in the ancestral amphibians was variable. *Ichthyostega* had seven on its hind limbs; *Acanthostega* had eight on its forelimbs and its hind limbs; and *Tulerpeton* had six digits on each limb (Coates 1996). The details of the adaptive radiation that led from predominantly aquatic amphibia to the true land animals are hidden in the Tournasian fossil gap between 354 and 339 million years ago. However, we know that primitive reptiles had five toes, and this trait was shared with their immediate amphibian ancestors. In addition to acquiring efficient limbs for terrestrial locomotion, the reptiles evolved a urinogenital system capable of producing an amniote egg; that is, an egg that could be laid on land because the shell and the amniotic membrane surround the developing embryo and prevent water loss. The amniote egg is also a trait of birds, but mammals have evolved a shell-less egg that is retained within the uterus and the fetus is nourished by a placenta.

If the genetic link between the urinogenital system and the limbs is indeed a primitive association, this may mean that most tetrapods with the primitive five-digit or pentadactyl limb will also have sexually dimorphic 2D:4D ratios. Much is known about the *Hox* gene control of digit and gonad formation in mammals from work with mice and rats (e.g., Herault et al. 1997; Peichel et al. 1997). This rodent system may be an ideal model with which to investigate the characteristics of the 2D:4D ratio. Further work is urgently required in order to establish whether mammalian and, in particular, rodent 2D:4D ratios are sexually dimorphic. If they are, then prenatal testosterone may be experimentally manipulated in order to establish its effect on 2D:4D ratio.

2D:4D in Primates and in Human Populations

What of differences in the 2D:4D ratio between nonhuman primates and humans and among human populations? There are few comparative data on 2D:4D ratio in monkeys and apes. Schultz (1924) was of the opinion that in all nonhuman primates the "fourth finger surpasses the second in length." In support of this he provided illustrations of fetal and adult hands of a platyrrhine (the howler monkey *Alouatta palliata*), a catarrhine (the colobus monkey *Colobus abyssinicus*), an orangutan (*Pongo pygmaeus*), and a chimpanzee (*Pan troglodytes*). Sorell (1968, 40) stated that nonhuman primates always have a digital formula of 3D > 4D > 2D > 5D > 1D, and he provided a photograph of the hand of a gorilla. There are other references in the literature to a long 4th digit and/or a low value of 2D:4D as characteristic of nonhuman primates or of an "atavistic" or "lower" human type (e.g., Ecker 1875). To my knowledge there are no published data to support these statements. Further work is needed to clarify the phylogenetic pattern of the 2D:4D ratio in primates.

It should be remembered that the *Hox* genes that control the formation of the gonads and the digits also influence the differentiation of the toes. There may be patterns of relative toe length that are sex-, population-, and species-dependent in humans and other primates. Schultz (1924) stated the relative lengths in apes as 3rd toe longer than 4th, which was longer than 2nd, and then 5th and finally 1st (3 > 4 > 2 > 5 > 1). The human fetus of the eighth and ninth week may show a formula of 3 > 4 > 2 > 1 > 5, which then changes in Caucasians to almost equal frequencies of 2 = 1 > 3 > 4 > 5 or 2 > 1 > 3 > 4 > 5 by the eighteenth week. I can find no data relating to sex differences in these formulae or in associations between 2D:4D ratio and relative toe length. In view of the putative relationships between 2D:4D and prenatal sex steroids and gonadal function, it is important to establish whether digit and toe ratios are linked.

Considering between-population differences in human 2D:4D ratio, Manning, Barley et al. (2000) have reported 2D:4D data from nine populations. Participants were measured directly from their right hands or from photocopies of their right hands. The mode of measurement did not affect the 2D:4D ratios. Samples were taken from the following populations:

the Liverpool area of northwest England (187 males and 210 females); the Granada area of southwest Spain (44 males and 52 females); central Poland around the city of Poznan (107 males and 105 females); southern Hungary in and around the city of Pecs (ethnic Hungarians, 19 males and 55 females; Hungarian Gypsies, 18 males and 45 females); Germany from the cities of Bielefeld, Hamburg, Hanover, Kassel, and Kiel (114 males and 121 females); a Zulu township of Natal (60 males and 60 females); a rural population in the south of Jamaica (78 males and 73 females); and a sample that was mainly from Helsinki in Finland (initially there were 24 males and 17 females, but this was later increased to 47 males and 54 females). An additional sample of Yanadi and Sugali people from Southern India was measured by Palla Venkatarama.

An inspection of data reveals strong differences in mean 2D:4D ratios between populations (see figure 1.7). High values of 2D:4D are present in the samples from Poland, Spain, and England; intermediate values in ethnic Hungarians, Hungarian Gypsies, Germans, and Indians; and low values in Zulus, Finns, and Jamaicans. We can see this clearly from the proportion of subjects per sample who have 2D:4D ratios of less than 0.999, i.e., toward the "male end" of the distribution. The proportions are

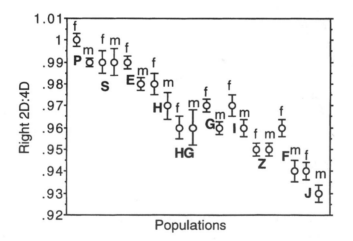

Figure 1.7. Differences in 2D:4D ratio of the right hand between populations and sexes in 10 cultures. P = Poland, S = Spain, E = England, H = Hungary, HG = Hungary Gypsy, G = Germany, I = India, Z = Zulu (South Africa), F = Finland, J = Jamaica. Sex is indicated by f = female and m = male. Substantial between-population differences are revealed. The Polish, Spanish, and English samples show high 2D:4D ratios; the German, ethnic Hungarian, Hungarian Gypsies, and Indians intermediate values of 2D:4D; the Zulu, Finnish, and Jamaican samples show low 2D:4D ratios. The mean ratios are rounded to the nearest 0.01.

as follows: Spain 66%, Poland 68%, England 68%, Hungary (ethnic Hungarians) 76%, India 77%, Germany 87%, Hungary (Gypsies) 91%, South Africa (Zulus) 93%, Finland 93%, Jamaica 97%. These proportions include both males and females. This means that many females in the Zulu, Finnish, and Jamaican samples have lower ratios than males within the Polish, English, and Spanish samples. Within populations there are the expected differences between the sexes; i.e., males tend to have lower 2D:4D ratios than females. However, the sex differences appear to be relatively small in comparison to the population differences. This impression is confirmed from the results of a two-factor ANOVA, which shows significant group and sex differences but with the former accounting for more of the total variance than the latter (populations $F = 27.30$, $p = 0.0001$; sex $F = 6.33$, $p = 0.01$). There is also a visual impression that the sex difference increases as the mean population 2D:4D ratio decreases. However, the interaction factor, which tests whether sex differences interact with population differences, was not significant ($F = 1.72$, $p = 0.13$). Any description of the ratio in terms of sexual dimorphism should stress that within a population the ratio in men tends to be lower than in women. Also, it is clear from these data that a model that seeks to explain the evolution of sex differences in 2D:4D ratio should encompass an explanation for population differences. It should be noted that 2D:4D ratio is not unique in showing both sex and ethnicity differences. For example, the supraorbital ridges are larger in men than in women and provide a valuable and reliable means of sexing a skull. However, the size of the supraorbital ridges in black females often exceeds those in Caucasian males (Knight 1991). This applies to other areas of the body. On average the bodily dimensions of women compared with men (percentage of male dimensions) is about 94% (e.g., stature 93.5%). However, in such traits as total arm length, upper arm length, and forearm length, women are smaller than expected (approximately 91.0%) relative to men. Many of these traits show both sex and ethnic differences (see comparisons between Caucasian and African Americans in Knight 1991, 116).

    With data from only ten populations we must exercise caution in deducing worldwide patterns. There is no simple dichotomy for example between black and Caucasian populations in these data and we do not as yet have samples from Oriental populations. Therefore the assertion of Schultz (1924, 158) that a long 4th digit relative to 2nd digit length is a characteristic of the black races only is not accurate. There is weak evidence of a curvilinear change in 2D:4D with latitude. At or near the equator 2D:4D ratios appear to be low, rising with an increase in latitude and then reducing in high latitudes ($y = 0.74 + 0.012x - 1.48E - 4x^2$,

$F = 5.39, p = 0.045$). Gruning (1886) has provided mean 2D:4D ratios for samples from Lithuania (males 0.95, females 0.96) and Latvia (males 0.94, females 0.97). The ratios were calculated from digit length measured from the metacarpo-phalangeal joint to the tip of the digit, and as such are not strictly comparable to data in figure 1.7. However, the means for both sexes are less than one and both populations are from quite high latitudes.

Effect Size of Sexual Dimorphism in 2D:4D

Statistical tests such as the t test may show significant differences between male and female 2D:4D ratios, but they do not give a readily understood measure of the strength of the differences. This is more appropriately indicated by the use of effect sizes. The effect size may be calculated from the difference in two means (in this case the male and female mean 2D:4D) divided by the square root of the weighted mean of their two variances (Cohen 1992). For example, in a sample of 238 Germans, the males ($n = 115$) had a mean 2D:4D of the right hand of 0.955 ± 0.03SD; while the females ($n = 123$) had a ratio of 0.973 ± 0.033. A t test showed a significant sex difference, $t = 4.56, p = 0.0001$. The effect size was:

$$0.973 - 0.955/[(123*0.03^2 + 115*0.03^2)/(123 + 115)]$$
$$= 0.018/0.032 = 0.56$$

Cohen (1992) suggested that effect sizes of 0.2, 0.5, and 0.8 can be regarded as small, medium, and large respectively. In this sample the sexual dimorphism in 2D:4D is therefore a medium effect size. Some samples show evidence of small effect sizes. For example, a Zulu sample of 120 participants showed a male mean 2D:4D of the right hand of 0.946 ± 0.036 with a sample size of 60. The female mean was 0.953 ± 0.036 with 60 subjects. This difference was not significant ($t = 1.13, p = 0.27$) and showed a small effect size of 0.19. Many samples of male and female 2D:4D ratio show sex-dependent differences with effect sizes ranging from small to medium.

Differences in Right- and Left-Hand 2D:4D?

In addition to sex and population differences there is one other pattern of expression of the 2D:4D ratio, i.e., differences between the right and left hands, which deserve a mention. Tanner (1990) has suggested that sexually dimorphic traits in general, and the 2D:4D ratio in particular, tend to be expressed in the "male form" more strongly on the right side of the body in men. The pattern is apparently reversed in females. If correct this would mean that 2D:4D ratio was lower in the right hand than the left in males and higher in the right hand than left in females. This assertion is not as improbable as it may appear at first sight. Paired organs do sometimes show directional asymmetry in their growth patterns. For example, in hermaphrodites, with one testis and one ovary, the ovary is more frequently found on the left (Mittwoch and Mahadevaiah 1980). Directional asymmetries of the testes and the breasts are also associated with sex-dependent cognitive patterns. Kimura (1994) has shown that men with right-larger testes and women with right-larger breasts score highly on tests that favor males, while those with a left-larger pattern score highly on female-favoring tests. With regard to the directional asymmetry of the 2D:4D ratio we may test this with data from the "cross-cultural" survey of Manning, Barley, et al. (2000). Measurements of right and left hands were available from seven populations: Poland, Spain, England, Hungary (ethnic Hungarians and Hungarian Gypsies), Germany, and Jamaica. In total there were 567 males and 661 females. The mean of the difference between the 2D:4D ratios of the right and left hands (D_{r-l}) in males was -0.001 ± 0.03 and in females it was 0.0002 ± 0.03. Negative male values and positive female values support Tanner's suggestion. However, the difference between the male and female mean D_{r-l} was not significant $(t = 0.92, p = 0.36)$. A two-factor ANOVA with Population (A) and Sex (B) showed no significant differences in D_{r-l} between populations $(F = 1.33, p = 0.24)$ or between sexes $(F = 0.45, p = 0.50)$ or in the interaction between A and B $(F = 0.41, p = 0.87)$. Therefore, there is little in the way of strong support for Tanner's suggestion. However, there are indications in some of the studies I report in later chapters that a low value of D_{r-l} is a strong correlate of traits that are more common in males. For example, in chapter 2, data from a sample of 56 men and 44 women attending an infertility clinic showed a lower mean value of D_{r-l} in men compared to women and a positive relationship between D_{r-l} and estrogen. Moreover, Marshall (2000) has found significant heritability for D_{r-l} in 41 father-child pairs $(h^2 = 0.35 \pm 0.20, t = 2.33, p = 0.03)$ but not in 64 mother-child pairs $(h^2 = -0.14 \pm 0.13, t = 1.15, p = 0.27)$. The father-child relationship suggests that the side of lowest 2D:4D ratio is not random in that it tends to be the same in male parents and their children. There may indeed be a tendency for low D_{r-l} in males and high D_{r-l} in females, but the dimorphism is an elusive one. On this point it could be relevant that correlations between 2D:4D ratio and sperm counts and the concentrations of various hormones in men and women have been found to be stronger in the right hand than in the left (Manning et al. 1998). This in part supports Tanner's suggestion that "male factors" find their strongest expression in the right hand.

Conclusions

The data discussed in this chapter suggest an overall picture of the expression of 2D:4D ratio as follows: (a) There is some evidence that a significant proportion of the variance in 2D:4D is determined in utero (probably by week 13 or 14); (b) it is sexually dimorphic (males have lower 2D:4D than females within the same population); and (c) there are substantial population and ethnic differences in 2D:4D that are of greater magnitude than the within-population sex differences. In order to determine why 2D:4D is sexually dimorphic, we must consider the prenatal factors that may be important in its origin. These factors are discussed in chapter 2.

Associations with Testosterone and Estrogen

The next important question to address is what factors determine the 2D:4D ratio. I think the hormonal evidence reviewed below suggests that the relative lengths of the 2nd and 4th digits are influenced prenatally by testosterone and estrogen concentrations. Testosterone appears to stimulate the prenatal growth of the 4th digit while estrogen promotes the growth of the 2nd digit. A low value of 2D:4D therefore indicates a uterine environment high in testosterone and low in estrogen and is characteristic of males. A high 2D:4D suggests low prenatal testosterone and high estrogen and is characteristic of females. However, the relationship between the 2nd to 4th digit ratio and prenatal steroidal hormones is far from being completely understood. In this chapter I discuss the available evidence.

Development of the Gonads

To understand how prenatal testosterone and estrogen may affect fetal digits, we must first consider the development of the gonads and the fetal production of steroid hormones (see Migeon and Wisniewski 1998 for a review of the process of sexual differentiation). Germ cells form in the yolk sac and migrate to the gonadal ridge at about five weeks of gestation. The wolffian ducts appear in the fourth week and the mullerian ducts during the sixth gestational week. If the embryo is male the wolffian ducts develop into the epididymis, vas deferens, and seminal vesicles. In females the mullerian ducts go on to form the fallopian tubes, uterus, and posterior portion of the vagina. The external genitalia form from the anterior end of the cloacal folds, and this tissue is bipotential until nine weeks of embryonic development.

Testis development involves three steps: (a) the appearance of Sertoli cells, which organize into seminiferous tubules, which surround the germ cells. The Sertoli cells produce a mullerian inhibiting substance (MIS) that prevents the further development of the female mullerian system. (b) The Leydig cells then appear and the fetal testis begins to produce testosterone; and (c) the germ cells differentiate into spermatogonia. Testosterone production starts at week 8 and peaks at week 13. Testosterone is essential for the further differentiation of the wolffian system and the fusion of

24

the urethral folds, growth of the scrotal area, and the formation of the penis from the genital tubercle. The precursor of testosterone is choles- terol. There are four enzymes required for its production. Further change in testosterone to dihydrotestosterone (a highly active form of testoster- one) occurs in the cells of the external genitalia.

In the absence of MIS from the Sertoli cells the mullerian system dif- ferentiates. Ovarian development consists of (a) the formation of oocytes; (b) folliculogenesis from the original bipotential gonad; and (c) the for- mation of endocrine cells. Estrogen is formed from testosterone by the action of aromatase, which is found in the fetal ovaries and the placenta. Aromatase in the placenta prevents maternal testosterone from diffusing to the fetus and fetal testosterone from virilizing the mother.

Digits, Testosterone, and Sperm Counts

The relationship between 2D:4D ratio and fetal testosterone is difficult to measure directly. There is evidence that 2D:4D ratio is fixed prenatally, and a relationship between adult 2D:4D ratio and testosterone may indi- cate a similar association in utero. In this section I address the prediction that low 2D:4D ratio, i.e., a more malelike ratio, is associated with high testosterone and high sperm counts. I use one-tailed tests when predicted relationships are indeed negative.

Relative finger length, particularly 2D:4D and 4th digit length adjusted for height, has been reported as being related to testosterone concentra- tion in adult men (Manning et al. 1998). The length of the 2nd and 4th digit of the right and left hands was measured in a sample of 131 patients (69 males and 62 females) attending an infertility clinic. Total serum tes- tosterone was assayed in a subsample of 58 men. Subjects with low 2D:4D (i.e., relatively long 4th digits) had more testosterone than participants with high 2D:4D (i.e., relatively short 4th digits), and this association was stronger in the right hand (right hand $b = -7.90$, $F = 5.02$, $p = 0.015$ one- tailed, adjusted for multiple tests $p = 0.03$, left hand $b = -6.10$, $F = 3.11$, $p = 0.04$ one-tailed, adjusted for multiple tests $p = 0.08$; see figure 2.1). Testosterone concentrations are negatively related to age and can be re- duced in obese men. A simultaneous multiple regression analysis with tes- tosterone as the dependent variable showed that 2D:4D of the right hand remained negatively related to hormonal level ($b = -6.93$, $t = 1.85$, $p = 0.035$ one-tailed), while age ($b = -0.01$, $p = 0.96$), weight ($b = -0.33$, $p = 0.37$), and height ($b = 0.81$, $p = 0.64$) were not associated with tes- tosterone concentrations.

Sperm counts have also been found to be associated with 2D:4D. Men with low 2D:4D or a more malelike ratio have more sperm in their

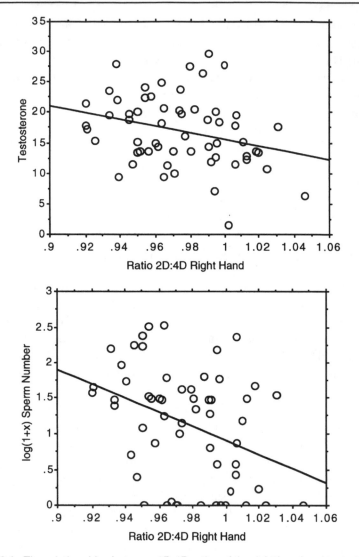

Figure 2.1. The relationships between 2D:4D ratios of the right hand and testosterone concentration and sperm numbers in 58 men attending an infertility clinic. The subjects with low 2D:4D or "malelike ratios" had higher testosterone levels and more sperm than subjects with high or "femalelike ratios."

ejaculates than men with a more femalelike ratio (Manning et al. 1998; right hand $b = -44.97$, $F = 8.59$, $p = 0.002$ one-tailed, adjusted for multiple tests $p = 0.004$; left hand $b = -25.69$, $F = 2.65$, $p = 0.055$ one-tailed, adjusted for multiple tests $p = 0.11$; figure 2.1). This relationship was independent of weight of the subject ($p = 0.002$ one-tailed). In the sample of 58 men there were 12 subjects with germ cell failure. That is, they produced no sperm or sperm that were inactive. These participants had high femalelike ratios in the right hand when compared to the men who produced motile sperm (germ cell failure males mean 2D:4D = 1.00 ± 0.005; males with motile sperm mean 2D:4D = 0.97 ± 0.004, $t = 2.11$, $p = 0.02$ one-tailed, adjusted for multiple tests $p = 0.04$). The left hand showed similar but nonsignificant differences (germ cell failure males mean 2D:4D = 0.98 ± 0.01; males with motile sperm mean 2D:4D = 0.96 ± 0.004, $t = 0.83$, $p = 0.21$ one-tailed). In the subsample with motile sperm ($n = 46$ men), there was evidence for relationships between 2D:4D ratios and sperm viability and progression, particularly for the right hand. Men with low 2D:4D ratios tended to have higher scores for sperm motility (right hand $p = 0.24$ one-tailed), average speed (right hand $p = 0.03$ one-tailed), percentage progressive sperm (right hand $p = 0.04$ one-tailed), and the Sperm Migration Test (right hand $p = 0.04$ one-tailed). These relationships were nonsignificant after adjustment for multiple tests. Further work is necessary to clarify the associations between the performance-related traits of sperm and 2D:4D ratios.

The relationships between 2D:4D ratio and testosterone and sperm counts appear to be dependent on the length of the 4th digit. The 4th digit adjusted for height of the subject (4D/height [m^2]) is positively related to both testosterone and sperm counts (see figure 2.2).

2D:4D Differences in Right and Left Hands

The associations between 2D:4D and sperm counts and testosterone were found to be strongest in the right hand. This may simply be a chance association. However, it does lend some support to Tanner's (1990) observation that the 2D:4D ratio is "more malelike" in the right hand of men than in the left. It may be the case that the digits of the right hand are more sensitive to androgens (Manning et al. 1998). If this is so the difference between the right and left 2D:4D ratio (D_{r-l} = right 2D:4D – left 2D:4D) should be lower in men than in women. This sample did in fact show such a sex difference in D_{r-l} (male mean = 0.01 ± 0.02; female mean = 0.02 ± 0.02; Mann-Whitney U test, Z-corrected for ties = 2.65, $p = 0.008$). An inspection of data suggests that male D_{r-l} is distributed bimodally (see figure 2.3). In support of this the distribution was found to be significantly platykurtosed. Platykurtosis in a sample suggests it is made up of two distributions with different means and similar variances (Zar 1984).

Men attending infertility clinics could be of normal fertility (often with partners with lowered fertility) or of mildly or severely compromised fertility (Wu 1983). The group of men with $D_{r-l} > 0.01$ may have reduced fertility. Although the latter group had lower mean sperm numbers per

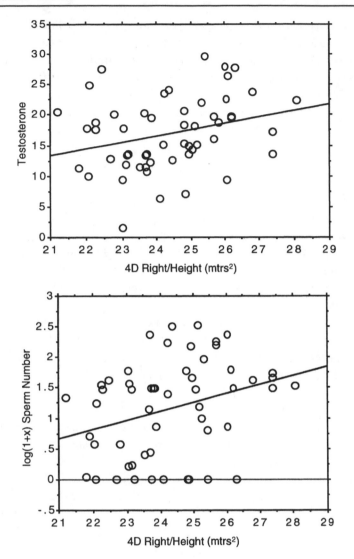

Figure 2.2. Men with long 4th digits adjusted for their height (4D/height [m²]) have more testosterone ($b = 1.06$, $F = 4.50$, $p = 0.04$) and higher sperm counts ($b = 0.15$, $F = 5.17$, $p = 0.03$) than men with short 4th digits adjusted for height.

ejaculate than the former, the difference was not significant ($D_{r-l} < 0.01$, mean sperm number $51.58 * 10^6$; $D_{r-l} > 0.01$, mean sperm number $42.22 * 10^6$; Mann-Whitney U test, Z-corrected for ties 0.42, $p = 0.67$). There was also a negative but nonsignificant correlation between testosterone and $\log (1 + x) D_{r-l}$ ($r = -0.08$, $F = 0.34$, $p = 0.56$) and between $\log (1 + x)$ sperm number and $\log (1 + x) D_{r-l}$ ($r = -0.18$, $F = 1.88$, $p = 0.18$). It

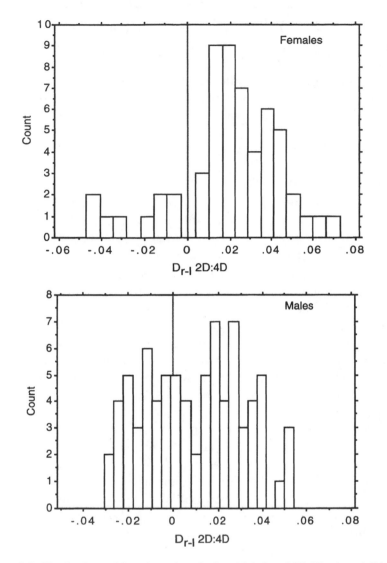

Figure 2.3. Distributions of female and male D_{r-l} (right hand 2D:4D minus left hand 2D:4D) in 62 women and 69 men attending an infertility clinic. Men have lower D_{r-l} values than women, and there is a suggestion of a bimodal distribution in men which shows significant platykurtosis (kurtosis = −0.96, SE = 0.55, Z = 1.92, p = 0.03). Platy-kurtosis in a sample suggests it is made up of two distributions with different means and similar variances. The bimodality in the male distribution may relate to a group of men with high or medium fertility (low D_{r-l}) and a group of low fertility men (high D_{r-l}).

seems, therefore, that D_{r-l} may be a negative indicator of androgenization, but it is not as strong as the 2D:4D ratio (see chapter 1). However, it should be noted that D_{r-l} is an asymmetry that is likely to increase with increasing prenatal androgen concentrations. This is because higher and higher testosterone concentrations will drive the 2D:4D ratio of the right hand lower and lower. The left hand may show a less-marked response. This means that D_{r-l} may be a powerful correlate of fetal androgenization in populations with low mean 2D:4D.

2D:4D and Hirsute Digits

These patterns of androgenization and 2D:4D are in adults, but 2D:4D is fixed before birth so that the associations may well represent relationships with in utero testosterone concentrations and morphogenesis and with the function of the testes that relate to prenatal conditions. With the differentiation of Leydig cells the male fetus begins to produce testosterone at about week 8 of development, and it is maximally produced in week 13 (Migeon and Wisniewski 1998). Relative digit length appears to be fixed by week 14 (Garn et al. 1975). Therefore, it is possible that testosterone may influence fetal digit length. If this is so we should find that all or some of the tissues of the 4th digit are liberally endowed with androgen receptors, while the other digits and especially the 2nd digits have fewer such receptors. We must wait for a detailed demonstration that this is so for cartilage and connective tissue. There is some circumstantial evidence that points to a high sensitivity to androgen in the dermis of the 4th digit. Look at the back of your fingers. The middle segments (phalanx 2 or P2) may have some hair on them. The presence of hair in this position is slightly more likely if you are male and much more likely on your 4th digit compared to your 3rd and 5th. It is very unlikely that you will find hair in this position on your 2nd digit. Furthermore, the 3rd or middle finger tends to be hairier than the 5th or little finger. Why this pattern? Hair growth in this position is dependent on testosterone and a metabolically active form of testosterone, dihydroxytestosterone (DHT). For example, P2 hair growth is more luxuriant in Kavango men than in men of the !Kung San from the same area of Namibia. Testosterone and DHT concentrations are higher in the former group compared to the latter, and within each group hair growth on P2 is positively related to androgen levels (Winkler and Christiansen 1993). In fact, growth of hair on P2 centers on the 4th digit and extends fieldlike to the 3rd, 5th, and finally the 2nd digit. Cartilage is not derived from the same tissue as the dermis. However, the androgen-dependent pattern of digit length is remarkably similar to that of hair growth. Hair is most likely on the 4th and 3rd digit and least likely on the 2nd. The 2D:4D ratio is sexually dimorphic but this also applies to the

2D:3D ratio. Both ratios are lower in men (i.e., longer 4th and 3rd digits) than in women (Phelps 1952). I therefore think it likely that most tissues in the 4th and 3rd digits are sensitive to androgen.

2D:4D and Correlates of Testosterone in Women

I have thus far assumed that prenatal exposure to testosterone is dependent largely on androgen produced by the fetal testes. Another source of testosterone, in both males and females, is from the adrenal glands, and the female fetus is exposed to androgen from this source. Fetal genes for testosterone production are inherited from the mother and father. Correlates of testosterone in mothers may therefore relate to fetal testosterone concentrations and to the 2D:4D ratio of their children. I will discuss two such correlates: (a) the 2D:4D ratio of mothers and (b) a proxy of adult testosterone (and estrogen) concentration, i.e., the ratio between waist and hip circumference.

A study of testosterone concentrations of fetuses and the 2D:4D ratios of their mothers has revealed a negative association. That is, high concentrations of fetal testosterone are found in the amniotic fluid of children of low 2D:4D ratio mothers (Lutchmaya, Baron-Cohen, and Manning, manuscript). The subjects were part of a longitudinal study of fetal testosterone and social-communicative development. Blood was obtained from routine amniocentesis tests performed at a mean gestational age of 17.06 ± 1.41 weeks. None of the amniocentesis tests showed an abnormality. The amniotic fluid was analyzed as a proxy for serum fetal testosterone (Finegan et al. 1991). Mothers and children (45 mother-infant pairs) attended a 24-month follow-up, and flat-bed scans of their hands were obtained. The images of the children's hands were often blurred due to movement, but most of the images from the mothers were of high quality. After discarding blurred scans, the sample sizes were 45 mothers and 19 children. Both mothers and children showed negative relationships between 2D:4D and fetal testosterone concentration. The association between 2D:4D left hand and testosterone was significant for mothers (see figure 2.4) but not for children ($b = -2.91$, $F = 0.77$, $p = 0.39$).

The WHR is a sexually dimorphic trait that becomes more obvious at puberty. Fat cell distribution in women and men is influenced by levels of sex hormones (Evans et al. 1983; Bjorntorp 1991). After puberty and under the influence of estrogen women tend to deposit fat peripherally (with the exception of the stomach) and on the buttocks and thighs (Garn 1957). Men, under the influence of testosterone, deposit fat in the abdominal region and on the shoulders and the nape of the neck (Vague et al. 1974). These patterns produce a gynoid or low WHR and an android or high WHR (Singh 1993). Among women there is considerable variation in

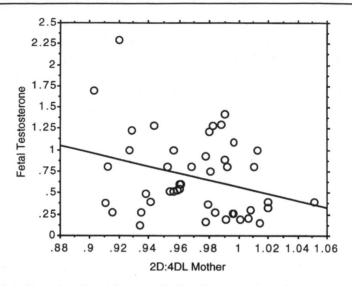

Figure 2.4. Mothers with malelike low 2D:4D ratios tend to have higher concentrations of testosterone in the amniotic fluid of their children than mothers with femalelike high 2D:4D ratio ($b = -4.03$, $F = 4.09$, $p = 0.02$, one-tailed, Bonferroni corrected for right-hand test $p = 0.04$).

WHR. Low WHR women have low testosterone and high estrogen levels, while high WHR women have high testosterone and low estrogen concentrations (Evans et al. 1983). There are considerable health and fertility implications for the WHR (Singh 1993). For example, in women increasing androgenicity, as reflected in a decrease in plasma sex hormone binding globulin capacity and an increase in free testosterone, is related to high WHR and an accompanying disruption in the homeostasis of the glucose-insulin balance (Kissebah et al. 1982; Evans et al. 1982; Evans et al. 1983). There is evidence in men for a preference for low WHR women (Singh 1993; Singh and Young 1995).

A recent study of Jamaican women has shown that their WHR is correlated with the 2D:4D ratio of their sons and daughters (see figure 2.5). As expected, if mother and fetus have genes in common for testosterone production, women with low WHR have high 2D:4D ratio children while more tubular women have low 2D:4D ratio children (Manning et al. 1999). There was no association between the WHR of mothers and D_{r-l} of their children.

Associated with these relationships is a suggestion that women with thick waists and high WHR have more sons than narrow-waisted women with low WHR (in an English sample, Manning et al. 1996; in a Texas sample, Singh and Zambarano 1997; and in a Jamaican sample, Manning et al. 1999). This may mean that women who have genes for high levels of testosterone also tend to have more sons than daughters. Such a possibility hints at potential conflict at the prenatal level. Genes for high prenatal testosterone concentrations may be advantageous if the fetus is male but disadvantageous if it is female. For example, the expression of genes for high testosterone in the female fetus could increase the chance of miscarriage. The action of such genes may be sexually antagonistic.

There is also evidence that the 2D:4D ratio of women and men is associated with their WHR. Firstly considering women, a sample of 185 English ($n = 92$) and Jamaican ($n = 93$) women was measured for 2nd and 4th digit length of the right and left hands and waist and hip circumference (Manning, Barley et al. 2000). There was a significant negative relationship between the 2D:4D ratio of the right hand and WHR; i.e., women with low 2D:4D ratio had a high waist:hip ratio (see figure 2.6). The left hand showed a negative nonsignificant association. The relationship in the right hand remained significant when ethnicity was controlled for (simultaneous multiple regression, right hand 2D:4D $b = -0.30$, $t = 2.30$, $p = 0.04$; ethnicity $b = 0.001$, $t = 0.47$, $p = 0.64$). This is evidence

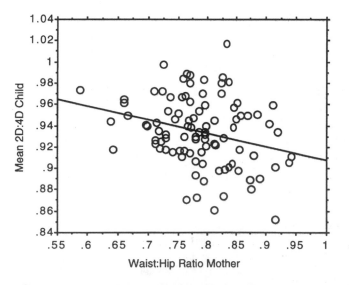

Figure 2.5. The relationship between waist:hip ratio (a trait positively associated with testosterone and negatively with estrogen) of Jamaican mothers and the mean 2D:4D ratio of their children ($n = 95$, left hand $b = -0.16$, $F = 8.72$, $p = 0.004$, Bonferroni adjusted for multiple tests $p = 0.008$; right hand $b = -0.10$, $F = 4.01$, $p = 0.048$). Women with low WHR had children with high 2D:4D ratio; that is, high estrogen and low testosterone was indicated in both mothers and children. High WHR is associated with low 2D:4D ratio thus showing evidence of low estrogen and high testosterone in both mothers and their children.

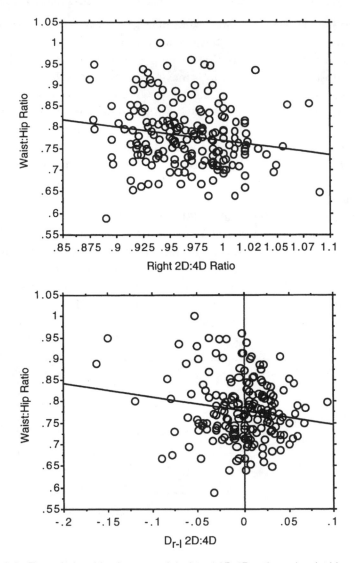

Figure 2.6. The relationships between right-hand 2D:4D ratio and waist:hip ratio and D_{r-l} and waist:hip ratio of 185 English ($n = 92$) and Jamaican ($n = 93$) women. Women with low 2D:4D ratio in the right hand and low D_{r-l} (ie indicating high prenatal testosterone) have high waist:hip ratios, while women with high 2D:4D ratio and high D_{r-l} (i.e., indicating low prenatal testosterone concentrations) have low WHR. WHR and 2D:4D, right hand $r = -0.18$, $F = 6.03$, $p = 0.02$, Bonferroni adjusted $p = 0.04$, left hand $r = -0.04$, $F = 0.31$, $p = 0.58$. WHR and D_{r-l} $r = -0.16$, $F = 4.71$, $p = 0.03$.

that women who have been exposed to high prenatal testosterone (i.e., those who have low 2D:4D) tend to have high WHR. The tendency is weak, but in this instance D_{r-l} also proved to be a significant negative correlate of WHR (figure 2.6). The relationship remained significant after controlling for ethnicity (D_{r-l} $b = -0.33$, $t = 2.29$, $p = 0.03$; ethnicity $b = 0.003$, $t = 1.62$, $p = 0.11$). Therefore, women with low 2D:4D in the right hand compared to the left also had high WHR. Secondly, considering men, a sample of 148 Caucasian men from the northwest of England were measured for 2D:4D and WHR. The mean age and WHR of the subjects was 64.86 ± 9.83 years and 0.92 ± 0.08. There was a nonsignificant negative association between 2D:4D and WHR (right hand $b = -0.31$, $F = 2.73$, $p = 0.10$; left hand $b = -0.05$, $F = 0.06$, $p = 0.81$). As with women there was also a significant negative association between D_{r-l} and WHR (see figure 2.7). These data provide further support for the suggestion that 2D:4D is negatively related to testosterone and positively related to estrogen. They also provide another indication that the right 2D:4D ratio is more sensitive to sex hormones than the left 2D:4D ratio.

Turning to the ventral surface of the hand, testosterone may have a prenatal influence on the complex pattern of ridges found on the digits and the palm. Asymmetries of ridge counts, i.e., differences in number of ridges between left and right hands, have been found to correlate with testosterone levels in adult men (Jamison et al. 1993). These dermatoglyphic patterns are fixed before the nineteenth week of pregnancy. Therefore their association with adult testosterone levels may well reflect relationships between prenatal testosterone and the formation of the epidermis and dermis of the digits (see chapter 1 for evidence from very low birth weight children). Overall the evidence is for the hand to be the site of a number of prenatally determined traits that are related to concentrations of testosterone in adults. It seems reasonable to assume that such traits are markers for uterine levels of testosterone.

2D:4D, Testosterone, and Population Differences

What then of testosterone and population and ethnic differences in 2D:4D ratio? I have argued that between-population differences in 2D:4D ratio are even larger than sex differences. If 2D:4D ratio is dependent on prenatal androgens, there should be evidence that testosterone also shows between-population differences in adults. There are indications from the literature that this is so. A comparison of the pedomorphic !Kung San of Tsumkwe, Namibia, with Kavango men of the Namibian/Angolan border area has shown significant differences in androgens (Winkler and Christiansen 1993). Serum concentrations of total testosterone, dihydrotestosterone, and salivary bioavailable non–SHBG-bound testosterone

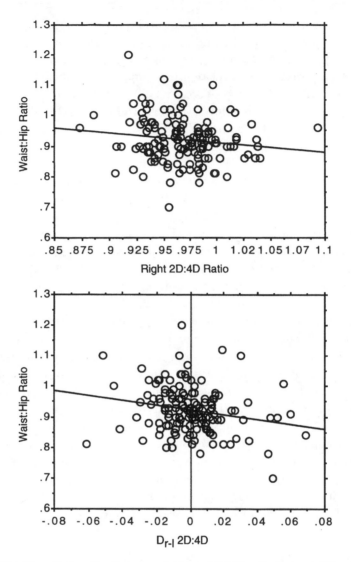

Figure 2.7. The relationships between right-hand 2D:4D ratio and waist:hip ratio and D_{r-l} and waist:hip ratio of 145 English men. Subjects with low 2D:4D ratio in the right hand and low D_{r-l} (i.e., indicating high prenatal testosterone) tended to have high waist:hip ratios (not significant for 2D:4D). WHR and 2D:4D (right hand $b = -0.31$, $F = 2.73$, $p = 0.10$, left hand $b = -0.05$, $F = 0.06$, $p = 0.81$); WHR and D_{r-l} ($b = -0.78$, $F = 6.26$, $p = 0.01$).

were all higher in Kavango men. Differences in testosterone levels have also been found between African Americans and Caucasians. In a sample of black and white college students in Los Angeles, mean total testosterone concentrations in black students were 19% higher than in whites and free testosterone levels 21% higher. Adjustment for age, weight, alcohol use, cigarette smoking, and prescription drug use reduced these differences to 15% and 13%, respectively. However, the ethnic differences in level of androgens remained statistically significant (Ross et al. 1986). Similar results were found by Ellis and Nyborg (1992) in a study of 525 black, 3,654 non-Hispanic white, and 200 Hispanic participants. The black subjects had higher mean testosterone concentrations than the Hispanic and non-Hispanic groups. There were no significant differences between Hispanics and non-Hispanic participants. There may also be significant within-Caucasian differences in concentrations of prenatal testosterone. Testosterone, vitamin D, and melanin compete for the same precursor, cholesterol (Bell et al. 1980). In areas with low levels of sunlight the synthesis of vitamin D is reduced. It may then be adaptive to reduce melanin production and therefore increase the synthesis of vitamin D. Reducing the production of melanin could also lead to an increase in the production of testosterone. There is indirect evidence that blond hair may be associated with high prenatal testosterone. Geschwind and Galaburda (1985a) have argued that the frequency of non–right-handedness is increased by high levels of in utero testosterone (see chapter 4 for evidence of an association between 2D:4D and left-hand preference). They found that in a sample of 986 nonblonds 76% were right-handed, 12% were ambidextrous, and 12% were left-handed. The corresponding figures for 131 blond-haired subjects were 56%, 28%, and 16% respectively. These observations are consistent with the possibility of high prenatal testosterone and low digit ratios in people of the northern latitudes.

Digits and Estrogen

Prenatal estrogen is derived from the action of aromatase in the placenta and from the maternal bloodstream. The 2D:4D ratio has been reported to be positively related to estrogen levels in a sample from an infertility clinic. This effect is independent of the influence of sex and is significant in the right hand ($p = 0.015$, one-tailed test, adjusted for multiple tests $p = 0.03$; Manning et al. 1998). That is, individuals with low malelike ratios in the right hand tend to have low levels of estrogen, and high femalelike ratios are related to high estrogen concentrations. This association suggests that in utero growth of the 2nd digit may be stimulated by estrogen. A significant positive association between D_{r-l} and estrogen is also seen

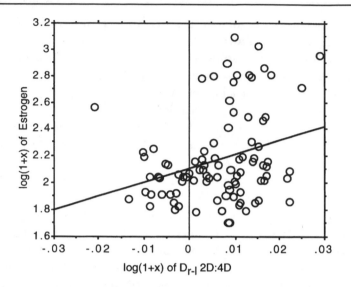

Figure 2.8. There are positive relationships between 2D:4D of the right hand minus 2D:4D of the left hand (D_{r-l}) and estrogen levels. Subjects with low D_{r-l} (a malelike trait) have lower estrogen than subjects with high D_{r-l} (a femalelike trait). The strength of the correlation with $n = 98$ is $r = 0.29$, $p = 0.004$.

in these data ($r = 0.29$, $p = 0.004$; figure 2.8). However, the relationship becomes nonsignificant after controlling for sex (multiple regression, D_{r-l} $b = 4.49$, SE $= 2.81$, $t = 1.60$, $p = 0.11$; sex [males $= 1$, females $= 2$] $b = 0.44$, SE $= 0.06$, $t = 7.95$, $p = 0.0001$).

In addition to positive relationships between 2D:4D and estrogen Manning et al. (1998) also found positive associations between 2D:4D ratios and luteinizing hormone (LH) in right and left hands of men and women (right hand $b = 10.26$, $F = 8.99$, $p = 0.002$ one-tailed, adjusted for multiple tests $p = 0.004$; left hand $b = 7.00$, $F = 3.85$, $p = 0.024$ adjusted for multiple tests $p = 0.049$). LH production in males is controlled by negative feedback by testosterone (Bell et al. 1980). Low 2D:4D in men is associated with both high testosterone and low LH in these data, an observation that is further evidence for the association between 2D:4D and testosterone. In females LH is controlled by both negative and positive feedbacks with estrogen depending on position in the menstrual cycle (Bell et al. 1980). In general LH concentrations are higher in females than in males; therefore, sex needs to be partialed out of the relationship between 2D:4D ratio and LH. A simultaneous multiple regression with LH the dependent variable showed that both 2D:4D of the right hand and sex were predictors of LH levels (2D:4D $b = 38.89$, $t = 2.27$, $p = 0.03$; sex $b = 3.54$, $t = 3.14$, $p = 0.002$). The 2D:4D of the right hand also remained a significant positive predictor of LH when the influence of sex, age, height, and weight were removed ($b = 8.49$, $t = 2.37$, $p = 0.02$). None of the remaining independent variables predicted LH concentrations. I interpret these data as indicating that low 2D:4D in men and women correlates with low LH concentrations and that high 2D:4D individuals tend to have high LH levels.

There is some evidence for estrogen receptors on fetal digits. Estrogen and progesterone treatment in the first trimester is associated with malformations of the genitalia in male children and also digit anomalies such as polydactyly, digit reduction, and fingerization of thumbs (Levy et al. 1973; Nora et al. 1976; Lorber et al. 1979). This overall picture suggests that exogenous prenatal estrogen may disrupt the action of *Hox* genes on developing genitalia and digits. That most of this deleterious effect is expressed in boys suggests that genes for the secretion of prenatal estrogen may have a sexually antagonistic effect; i.e., they are advantageous in the female fetus but not in the male fetus.

Conclusions

The data concerning the nature of the association between 2D:4D and prenatal steroid hormones are indirect. I think the evidence is quite persuasive, but at present it is not possible to say with complete confidence that testosterone facilitates the growth of the 4th digit and that estrogen enhances the growth of the 2nd digit. We need more direct evidence to settle the matter. Data from adults suggest that low 2D:4D, low D_{r-l}, and long 4th digit controlled for height are related to a number of variables, which include high sperm counts, high testosterone, and low estrogen. These associations may well reflect prenatal influences of testosterone. In general it seems that low 2D:4D is the most reliable of the predictors of hypermasculinization, and it is this trait that provides the most convincing evidence of a prenatal origin. There are a large number of instances, from a large number of different fields of inquiry, in which prenatal testosterone and/or estrogen have been implicated in the etiology of traits. In succeeding chapters I provide evidence that a whole suite of traits and disease predispositions are correlated with 2D:4D.

A note on statistical treatment: The main trait addressed in this book is 2D:4D. In general I consider index trait (e.g., reproductive success, running speed) associations with both right and left hand 2D:4D ratios. Adjustments for multiple tests are made. One-tailed tests are only used when there is a clearly predicted direction to the association. For example, low 2D:4D is associated with high sperm counts and high testosterone; therefore, a negative association may be predicted between 2D:4D and lifetime reproductive success in men. Mean 2D:4D ratio is not independent of right and left hand ratios and is not in general considered. In a similar way D_{r-l} is not independent of right and left 2D:4D, and the associations of 2D:4D or D_{r-l} with an index trait such as running speed are also not independent. For completeness I have reported associations between D_{r-l} and index traits, but with this non-independence in mind I do not place emphasis on this trait. Fourth digit length corrected for body size (height) is a correlate of 2D:4D and probably associated with androgenization, but we have no evidence as to when this trait is fixed. For this reason it is of less interest than 2D:4D. I discuss the trait in relationship to aggression in boys (where 2nd digit measurements were not available) and in the study on male depression where there are suggestive but non-significant associations with 2D:4D ratio and the index trait.

CHAPTER 3

Assertiveness, Status, Aggression, Attractiveness, and the Wearing of Rings

I have presented evidence in the previous chapter that the 2D:4D ratio, the difference between right and left hand 2D:4D (D_{r-l}), and the length of the 4th digit adjusted for height may be correlates of prenatal and adult testosterone concentration. If testosterone is associated with 2D:4D ratio, is there any evidence that low 2D:4D ratio and/or long 4th digits are associated with assertiveness, status, and aggressive behavior? If so, the relative lengths of digits may also be used by females to assess the competitiveness of males. High status and wealth tend to be more highly valued by women than by men when making mate choices, and this effect is found across cultures (Buss 1985). It may be that some women perceive low 2D:4D ratios, or perhaps more likely, long 4th digits, as being attractive.

Assertiveness, Status, and Aggression

Aggression may be viewed as hostile behavior motivated by fear or frustration, a desire to produce fear or flight in others, or a tendency to push forward one's own ideas or interests (Reber 1985). This is a wide definition, which may include assertiveness in arguing a viewpoint through mild verbal aggression to violent physical aggression. An increase in status and wealth may be important payoffs for aggression. There is considerable uncertainty whether testosterone has a causal role in aggression (Archer 1991), and other hormones such as cortisol may be equally or more important (Raine 1993). In view of this uncertainty it may be instructive to examine whether the 2D:4D ratio or the length of the 4th digit adjusted for height are correlated with any forms of aggression including assertiveness, measures of status, verbal aggression, and physical aggression.

Assertiveness

Glenn Wilson (1983) has considered the relationship between assertiveness and 2D:4D ratio in women. He pointed out that 2D:4D was sexually dimorphic and that masculinity femininity of social behavior may follow similar lines across a range of ratios in women. In order to test this idea he designed a questionnaire for a national British newspaper entitled

"Changing Women in the 1980's." Within the questionnaire there were two questions which related to assertiveness and finger length. One asked the participants to classify themselves as "assertive or competitive," "fairly average," or "gentle and feminine" compared with other women. In another part of the questionnaire they were asked to measure the length of each finger in the left hand from the "lower wrinkle" to the tip excluding the fingernail.

There were 985 participants who gave "believable" measurements, i.e., within the expected range of finger length. The sample was divided into subjects with 2nd digit shorter than 4th, 2nd equal to 4th, and 2nd longer than 4th. Of the women with 2nd digits shorter than 4th, 31% described themselves as assertive or competitive whereas the proportion was 25% in the women with 2nd digits longer than 4th. The figure for participants with 2D = 4D was 29%. A Chi-Square analysis showed the differences to be significant at the 5% level.

The relationship between self-reported assertiveness and low 2D:4D was weak but nevertheless significant because of the size of the sample. However, it should be noted that the sample was probably not representative of population norms for 2D:4D. There were 648 subjects with 2D:4D less than 1, 70 with 2D:4D = 1, and 267 with 2D:4D greater than 1. For some reason the nature of the readership and/or the completion of the questionnaire has lead to a sample of participants with an excess of "male-type" ratios.

Wilson suggested his results had similarities with those of Schlegel (1975), who compared sexual dimorphism in the structure of the pelvis with intrasex measures of dominance and aggression. In Schlegel's data women with malelike narrow pelvic outlets tended to be more dominant and aggressive relative to women with wide pelvic outlets. Men with a broad pelvis were more feminine in personality than men with a narrow pelvis. Sexual dimorphisms in the pelvis can be traced back to the prenatal period. Schlegel's study may indeed be evidence of an in utero influence on gender differences. There are similarities between these findings and those of Kimura and Carson (1995). In this work the sexually dimorphic trait was dermatoglyphic ridge counts. The overall count is higher in males than females. Both sexes have higher right-hand than left-hand counts, but there is a greater proportion of right-hand greater than left counts in males compared to females. Kimura and Carson found that subjects of both sexes with right greater than left ridge counts scored higher on male-favoring tests. Those with left greater than right asymmetry scored higher on female-favoring tests. The number of dermal ridges is fixed by the fourth month of fetal development (Holt 1968). These correlations suggest that intellectual pattern is influenced by prenatal factors.

Status

Testosterone may be a factor in drive, competitiveness, and recovery rates from muscular activity. However, high levels of prenatal testosterone may also predispose to dyslexia and poor verbal ability. In westernized societies it is not clear whether or how 2D:4D would be related to the acquisition of resources, and therefore to deprivation scores. Manning and Bundred (manuscript) examined the relationship of 2D:4D to socio-economic status in a sample of 210 patients (160 men and 50 women) attending a cardiac rehabilitation center in the Wirral area of northwest England. Age is likely to affect deprivation scores in that people may tend to accumulate wealth with increasing age. The mean age of the sample was 63.12 ± 10.30 years, and the range was from 29 to 90 years. The Townsend deprivation score (Townsend et al. 1988) was used as a measure of socioeconomic status, and scores were accessed from postal codes. Townsend scores are a negative index of deprivation. They are calculated for postal code areas and are derived from four estimates of material deprivation—unemployment, nonownership of a car, nonowner occupation of houses, and household overcrowding. The scores in this sample ranged from minus 5 (the most affluent) to 10 (the least affluent) with a mean of 0.24 ± 3.61. We found a significant negative association between 2D:4D ratio and Townsend score in the right hand, but not the left hand of men. That is, a low 2D:4D in the right hand of males was associated with low socioeconomic status (see figure 3.1). Age was also associated with deprivation scores. Older men had higher socioeconomic status than younger men ($b = -0.06, F = 6.21, p = 0.01$). A simultaneous multiple regression analysis showed that low right-hand 2D:4D predicted high deprivation scores independent of age (2D:4D $b = -20.44, t = 2.70, p = 0.008$; age $b = -0.07, t = 2.98, p = 0.003$). D_{r-l} may be a negative correlate of prenatal testosterone. As expected we found that male D_{r-l} was negatively associated with Townsend scores, i.e., low D_{r-l} or right 2D:4D lower than left was related to high deprivation scores ($b = -17.36, F = 4.11, p = 0.04$). There was no association between 4th digit length divided by height and socioeconomic levels ($b = 4.61, F = 0.12, p = 0.73$). In the female sample there was no evidence of an association between right- and left-hand 2D:4D and Townsend scores. Both right- and left-hand 2D:4D showed a very weak positive association with deprivation scores (right hand $b = 0.25$, $F = 0.0003, p = 0.99$; left hand, $b = 3.15, F = 0.05, p = 0.82$).

I conclude from these preliminary data that low 2D:4D may indeed be related to high deprivation in men. It is of interest to know how widespread this relationship is. Cultures that stress the utility of male:male physical aggression and manual labor in the acquisition of resources may show relationships between high 2D:4D ratio and deprivation.

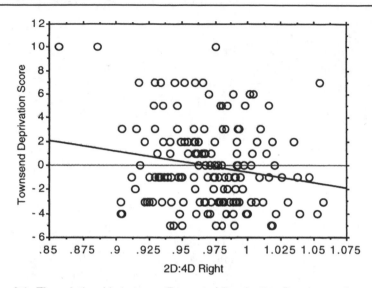

Figure 3.1. The relationship between Townsend Deprivation Score or socioeconomic status and the 2D:4D ratio of the right hand in 160 men. High Townsend scores indicate high levels of deprivation. The association was significant for the right hand ($b = -17.44$, $F = 5.16$, $p = 0.02$, Bonferroni corrected $p = 0.04$) and was independent of age ($p = 0.008$). There was no significant relationship in the left hand ($b = 1.25$, $F = 0.02$, $p = 0.88$). The association suggests that low 2D:4D in the right hand is correlated with high deprivation in men.

Aggression

Aggression, particularly physical aggression, is more frequent among human males than females and more common among young males than old males (Olweus et al. 1980). Some studies have found significant positive associations between testosterone and aggressive and criminal behavior (e.g., Olweus et al. 1980; Gladue 1991; Dabbs et al. 1995; and Banks and Dabbs 1996), but others have reported negative relationships (e.g., Meyer-Bahlburg et al. 1974, and reviews by Archer 1991, 1994). Depression in men has been reported as positively related to 4th digit length (and to a lesser extent 3rd) corrected for height (Martin et al. 1999). It may be that high prenatal testosterone could affect the developing brain predisposing it to depression and also to a tendency to a loss of control leading to aggression. Manning and Wood (manuscript) have investigated the relationship between 4th digit length corrected for height and aggression in boys ages 12 to 17.

The sample consisted of 150 boys recruited from the Liverpool area. All participants were from a single school recruiting from a catchment area that includes a wide range of socioeconomic groups. Age was recorded, and height and weight measured. The study was designed to address issues relating to aggression in teen-age boys. Unfortunately, the length of the 2nd digit was not measured, and we are therefore unable to relate 2D:4D to aggression in these data. The lengths of the 4th and 3rd digits of the right and left hands were measured. The means for age, height, and weight of the subjects were 13.44 ± 1.58 years, 1.68 ± 0.12 m, and 55.25 ± 11.00 kg respectively. The aggression questionnaires were completed by the participants after the measurements were made. All subjects were informed that the study concerned the association between morphological traits and aggression. The questionnaire was taken from the Olweus Multifaceted Aggression Inventory, which was designed for preadolescent and adolescent boys (Olweus et al. 1980). It consisted of two sections of five questions relating to verbal and physical aggression (see table 3.1). Each item was scored on a five-point scale (1: "I disagree strongly" to 5: "I agree strongly"). The questions and scales have been peer-validated and shown to have high internal consistencies (Olweus et al. 1980; Archer et al. 1995). Totals per subject for each scale were calculated and the sample means were verbal aggression 15.17 ± 2.81 and physical aggression 16.16 ± 3.27.

There were significant positive relationships between the length of the right and left 4th digit (divided by height [meters^2]) and total score for physical aggression per subject. The relationships were stronger for the right hand than for the left hand (see figure 3.2). That is, boys with long 4th digits adjusted for height reported more physical aggression compared with participants with short 4th digits. There was no significant pattern between 4th digit length and verbal aggression (right 4th digit, $b = -2.78, F = 1.52, p = 0.22$; left 4th digit, $b = -2.49, F = 1.33, p = 0.25$). The relationship between the length of the 4th digit of the right hand and

Table 3.1. Verbal and physical agression scales from the Olweus Multifaceted Aggression Inventory

Verbal Aggression (toward adults)
1. When an adult is unfair to me, I get angry and protest.
2. When an adult tries to take my place in a line, I firmly tell him it is my place.
3. When a teacher criticizes me, I tend to answer back and protest.
4. When a teacher has promised we will have some fun, but then changes his or her mind, I protest.
5. When an adult tries to boss me around, I resist strongly.

Physical Aggression (toward peers)
1. When a boy starts fighting with me, I fight back.
2. When a boy is nasty with me, I try to get even with him.
3. When a boy teases me, I try to give him a good beating.
4. I fight with other boys at school.
5. I really admire the fighters among the boys.

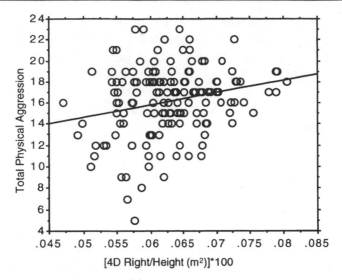

Figure 3.2. The relationship between Total Physical Aggression scores on the Olweus Scale and the length of the right 4th digit corrected for height (meters^2). The independent variable has been multiplied by 100 in order that variation in the scale can be seen. The relationship was significant for the right and left hands (right 4th digit, $b = 7.55$, $F = 8.62$, $p = 0.004$; left 4th digit, $b = 6.03$, $F = 5.91$, $p = 0.02$). There were no significant relationships between 4th digit length and verbal aggression. Reported physical aggression increases with an increase in 4th digit/height (meters^2). The sample was 150 Liverpool boys between the ages of 12 and 17.

physical aggression remained significant after adjustment for multiple tests ($p = 0.02$).

Factors other than prenatal testosterone concentrations are likely to influence physical aggression scores. A multiple regression analysis with dependent variable total physical aggression score per participant and independent variables 4th and 3rd digit length of the right hand, age, height, and weight showed that the length of the 4th digit remained a significant predictor of physical aggression. None of the remaining variables was significantly associated with physical aggression (see table 3.2). I con-

Table 3.2. Relationships between Olweus scores of physical aggression and variables

Trait	beta	SE	t	p
4th digit length	3.58	1.78	2.01	0.04
3rd digit length	−1.81	1.71	1.06	0.29
Age	−0.13	0.31	0.43	0.67
Height	−3.60	1.98	0.70	0.48
Weight	−0.04	0.04	0.83	0.41

clude from these data that 4th digit length adjusted for height is positively associated with measures of physical aggression in boys.

Attractiveness

If status and aggression are related to long 4th digits, then there may be a similar relationship between 4th digit length and sexual attractiveness. David and Brannon (1976) have pointed out that boys identify four general imperatives: avoid typical female behavior, achieve success, do not be dependent on anyone else, and be aggressive. Sadalla et al. (1987) reported four experiments that tested the relation between behavioral markers of dominance and the heterosexual attractiveness of males and females. They found that dominance behavior increased the attractiveness of males but had no effect on the attractiveness of females. The relationship between dominance and sexual attractiveness was found to be independent of likability when dominance level was manipulated. Mueller and Mazur (1997) obtained facial dominance ratings of a cohort of military officers who were graduates in 1950 of the U.S. Military Academy at West Point. High facial dominance ratings predicted rank attainment at the Academy and also final rank attainment. For men with discordant performance and dominance rating there was evidence that a dominant facial appearance was a handicap for promotion. Professional success influenced fitness. Generals had 3.67 children compared to a mean of 3.02 children for other officers ($p < 0.001$). The difference resulted from one parity progression to a third child. We do not yet know whether 4th digit length corrected for height correlates with ratings of facial dominance. If it does, then the hands of men with relatively long 4th digits may be rated as more attractive than the hands of men with short 4th digits.

Women value status, dominance, and resources in potential mating partners (Buss 1985). Men remain fertile for much of their adult lives, and this means that age-dependent accumulation of wealth can be used by males to maximize their lifetime reproductive fitness. Some women may, of course, simply choose to pair with older men with status and wealth. However, there may be disadvantages to this strategy, e.g., if the accumulation of harmful mutations in sperm is age-dependent. A trait that predicts future success in male-male competition for resources will be of interest to women and might be incorporated into mate-choice judgments. It seems unlikely that potential mates can assess 2D:4D ratio by simply looking at a hand or by "holding hands." However, finger length is a trait that is more readily estimated. Finger length and other aspects of the hands are likely to be correlated with variables that are important in mate choice, such as height and weight. The relative importance of such traits in perceptions of attractiveness has been considered by Manning and Crone (manuscript).

Ratings were made of photocopies of the ventral and dorsal surfaces of the hands. In all cases the quality of the photocopy was such that for palms the proximal crease at the base of the digits could be seen, and for the back of the hand the creases around the knuckles were visible. The right hands of 60 men and 91 women were photocopied. Subjects were asked to remove all rings. The height, weight, and age of the subjects was recorded. The length of the 2nd and 4th digits was measured from the basal crease of the finger to the tip. The photocopies were rated by a total of 20 raters (10 men and 10 women), and raters were allocated randomly so that 5 men and 5 women rated each subject. The hands were rated on a seven-point scale for sexiness, attractiveness, assertiveness, and intelligence. A rating of one was least sexy and seven most sexy. Raters were informed of the sex of the subject but were given no other information. For each subject means of ratings for same-sex raters and different-sex raters were calculated for ventral and dorsal photocopies. There were therefore four mean ratings per subject.

We are most concerned here with the ratings for sexiness and attractiveness. For both men and women digit length was positively related to both attributes; i.e., longer fingers were considered more sexy and attractive. The slope for the 4th digit was steeper than the slope for the 2nd. In men and women the weight of the subject was negatively related to sexiness and attractiveness; i.e., light individuals were considered more sexy and attractive. In men only height was positively related to both sexiness and attractiveness; i.e., tall men were rated more highly. In women only young subjects were rated more sexy and attractive.

Simultaneous multiple regression analyses were performed, controlling for sex of rater and dorsal/ventral view of the hand. It was found that long 4th fingers were significantly associated with perceptions of attractiveness and sexiness in both men and women. This rating was independent of potential confounding factors such as the length of the 2nd digit, height, weight, and age of the subject. The length of the 2nd digit was not significantly correlated with sexiness/attractiveness ratings. Negative relationships with sexiness/attractiveness were found for men and women for weight and for women only for age. That is, the hands of thin men and women and young women were rated as more sexy and attractive than those of heavier men and women and older women. Height was positively associated with attractiveness/sexiness for male subjects; i.e., the hands of tall men were rated higher than those of short men (see table 3.3). It appears that the factors that control 4th digit length, weight, height (in men only), and age (in women only) can affect perceptions of the attractiveness or sexiness of the hands.

Table 3.3. Predictors of sexiness in the right hand of males and females

	β Coefficient	St Error	Value	p
Males Rated for Sexiness				
2nd Digit	0.005	0.02	0.24	0.81
4th Digit	0.055	0.02	2.64	**0.009**
Height	0.016	0.01	2.40	**0.02**
Weight	−0.01	1.97	3.19	**0.002**
Age	−0.01	0.01	1.70	0.09
Sex Rater	−0.22	0.09	2.47	**0.01**
Palm/Back	0.007	0.09	0.07	0.941
Females Rated for Sexiness				
2nd Digit	−0.01	0.02	0.80	0.424
4th Digit	0.051	0.02	2.80	**0.005**
Height	0.003	0.01	0.37	0.713
Weight	−0.02	1.97	4.81	**0.001**
Age	−0.01	0.01	2.44	**0.015**
Sex Rater	−0.77	0.08	10.07	**0.001**
Palm/Back	−0.12	0.08	2.47	**0.014**

A long 4th digit may correlate with high testosterone levels in both men and women. It may therefore be associated with fertility in men. In women high testosterone is unlikely to correlate with fertility, but it may indicate high sex drive, an increased tendency to produce sons, and to have sons with a superior vascular system (see chapter 6). It is unclear why preferences for light women and men and tall men are adaptive. However, fluctuating asymmetry (FA), a negative correlate of phenotypic quality, has been reported to be low in tall men (Manning 1995) and light women (Manning 1995; Hume and Montgomerie 2001). There is also evidence from a Polish study that tall men are more likely to be married than short men and to have more children than short men (Pawlowski et al. 2000). A significant negative association between age and ratings of attractiveness was expected for women, as age is negatively associated with female fertility.

Multiple regression analyses of ratings for assertiveness showed few significant relationships. However, in women long 4th digits were rated as belonging to more assertive subjects ($p = 0.04$). This is of interest, as women with low or male-type 2D:4D ratios (i.e., relatively long 4th digits) report more assertiveness than women with high or female-type 2D:4D ratios (Wilson 1983). Ratings for intelligence showed significant correlations with height (positive relationship, $p = 0.03$) and weight (negative,

$p = 0.0004$) in men, and 4th digit length (positive, $p = 0.0001$), weight (negative, $p = 0.0001$), and age (negative, $p = 0.03$) in women.

Our findings that long 4th digits, but not 2nd digits, are rated as sexy and attractive in both men and women have implications for patterns of pairing in human populations. In general, people pair assortatively for most morphological traits; tall people assort with tall, short with short, etc. This overall tendency is rather weak but nevertheless often significant in samples of one or two hundred pairs of individuals. Digit length is no exception to this pattern of positive assortment. What of the 2D:4D ratio? A sample of 221 Liverpool couples showed positive associations between male and female 2nd digit ($b = 0.15$, $F = 4.56$, $p = 0.02$) and the 4th digit ($b = 0.18$, $F = 6.96$, $p = 0.001$), with the 4th digit showing the stronger association. There was also a rather weak but significant positive assortment pattern with mean 2D:4D ratio of the right and left hand ($b = 0.15$, $F = 4.58$, $p = 0.03$; see figure 3.3).

Such a pattern may result if long 4th digits are positively associated with attractiveness scores in men and women, and attractiveness itself shows positive assortment. We should not overemphasize the strength of the effect, but one implication of this is that populations may also show positive assortment for testosterone and estrogen concentrations. This could lead

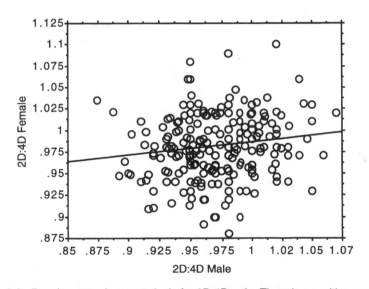

Figure 3.3. People may pair assortatively for 2D:4D ratio. There is a positive associa-tion between mean 2D:4D of sexual partners ($b = 0.15$, $F = 4.58$, $p = 0.03$). The effect is weak. However, it could lead to an increase in the numbers of individuals at the ex-tremes of the distribution of hormonal concentration, i.e., those with high testosterone, low estrogen, and low testosterone, high estrogen.

to an increase in the tails of the distribution for these two traits, i.e., more offspring with high and low hormone levels.

The Wearing of Rings

It is a remarkable coincidence that the 4th digit is associated with testosterone concentrations and sperm counts and is also the digit that is used to mark marital status in many cultures. Married women and men often wear a ring on their 4th digit, hence the common term *ring finger*. This custom dates back to at least Roman times. Laverack (1979) has suggested that its origins may lie in the early belief that a nerve, vein, or artery runs directly from the 4th digit to the heart. That is the organ which was judged to be the seat of the emotions. An alternative explanation is that the ring finger is less often used than the rest and cannot be extended alone. This property may protect the ring from damage (Laverack 1979). I can find no anatomical data to support the first contention, and the second suggestion does not explain why a ring should be worn in the first place. I suggest a third alternative. The ornamentation of the 4th digit indicates not only the wearers' marital status but also their commitment to their union. If this is so, rings should be displayed more frequently by individuals whose partners have high fertility or fitness.

Manning (manuscript) has examined this hypothesis in a sample of 79 married couples. The participants were recruited in Liverpool from adult education classes and social clubs. There was no noticeable socioeconomic bias in the sample. All couples had been married for a minimum of five years and had at least one child. The participants were told that this was a research project concerned with body measurements related to numbers of offspring. No measurements were made in the subjects' homes. This meant that all had to travel in public to the measurement sessions. Of the 79 couples there were 56 (71%) women who wore a ring or rings on their 4th digit and 23 (29%) men. Wedding rings are worn on the left hand, therefore measurements were made of the 2nd and 4th digits of the left hands. There was no evidence that the mean 4th digit length differed in women who wore rings and those who did not (with rings 72.3 ± 3.89 mm; without rings 71.46 ± 5.04 mm, $t = 0.81$, $p = 0.42$). This was also the case in the male sample (with rings 80.09 ± 4.00 mm; without rings 78.05 ± 5.94 mm, $t = 1.44$, $p = 0.15$). The prediction was that women wearing a ring on their 4th digit would have partners who had lower 2D:4D ratios than partners of participants who did not wear a ring on their 4th digits. There was some evidence to support this. The mean 2D:4D ratio of the husbands of women who were wearing rings was 0.97 ± 0.03. The mean 2D:4D ratio of the men whose wives were not wearing their wedding ring was 0.98 ± 0.04. This difference was significant in a one-tailed test ($t = 1.89$, $p = 0.03$). There was no evidence for any difference in the 2D:4D ratio of the partners of the men (with rings 0.99 ± 0.04; without rings 0.99 ± 0.03, $t = 0.12$, $p = 0.91$). The effect in the female sample was weak, and the work needs to be repeated. However, this is evidence that married women may advertise their commitment to their marriage by wearing or not wearing a ring on their 4th digit. It is possible that a nonornamented 4th digit could indicate to males an increased probability of extra-pair copulations (EPCs). The same situation does not apply to males. This is to be expected because sexual selection acts differently on females and males. Females are constrained by the high cost of eggs, pregnancy, and subsequent suckling and infant care so that their maximum number of offspring is low. They therefore invest heavily in the fitness of their offspring. Women may maintain marriages to men who are of low phenotypic and genotypic quality but who are able to provide resources for them and their children. EPCs with men of high phenotypic and genotypic quality may be expected in many such unions. Men produce low-cost sperm and are able to father large numbers of offspring given large numbers of partners. They are therefore selected to maximize their number of children both within and without their partnerships. High rates of EPCs in males may be related to their phenotypic and genotypic quality and not to the fertility of their partners.

Conclusions

I have presented evidence that 2D:4D ratio, D_{r-l}, and 4th digit length adjusted for height are related to a suite of traits that include assertiveness, status, male physical aggression, perceptions of attractiveness, patterns of assortative mating, and female ornamentation of the 4th digit. These aspects of sexual selection are likely to be associated in some way with fitness. I will now discuss the association of the 2D:4D ratio with lifetime reproductive success.

CHAPTER 4

Reproductive Success and Sexually Antagonistic Genes

I have discussed evidence that indicates 2D:4D ratios are lower in men than women, show significant differences between populations, are negatively related to sperm counts and testosterone concentrations, are positively associated with estrogen, and show relationships with status, and that the length of the 4th digit adjusted for height shows positive associations with physical aggression and perceptions of attractiveness of hands. Given these relations I now ask whether 2D:4D ratios are predictors of direct fitness, i.e., measures of reproductive success.

In human societies the number of offspring produced by an individual is likely to be influenced by many factors. These include the economic value of children (Harris 1989), rates of infant mortality (Lopreato and Yu 1988), one's own fertility, the fertility of one's partner or partners, the desire for children, and the effectiveness of available birth-control techniques. Some of these are group- and subgroup-specific, e.g., the economic value of children and infant mortality. These and other factors presumably result in differences in numbers of children between groups. Within-group variance in offspring number is likely to be influenced in part by individual fertility. Of course, in westernized societies there may be many couples who are fertile but who by choice produce few or no offspring. However, those who suffer from some degree of infertility may have considerable difficulty in having, say, four or five children. Therefore, it is possible that 2D:4D ratio may correlate with numbers of children, and more importantly numbers of children independent of age of individual. Before considering the relationship between 2D:4D and reproductive success, it is important to understand the kind of selection pressures operating on genes controlling prenatal testosterone and estrogen exposure. I think these selection pressures may be best understood within the context of sexually antagonistic genes.

Sexually Antagonistic Genes

Consider a man who has experienced high testosterone and low estrogen exposure in utero. It would increase his fitness if his sons shared these traits, and given some heritability of prenatal hormone production, it is to be expected that they will. They may therefore make many grand-children

53

for him. However, what of his daughters? Genes inherited from their father may cause them to produce high testosterone and low estrogen in utero. High levels of androgen could compromise the development of the female reproductive system and therefore reduce the fitness of his daughters. Similarly, a woman who has experienced low testosterone and high prenatal exposure to estrogen may produce fertile daughters but low-fertility sons. In such a situation modifiers of genes controlling in utero testosterone and estrogen exposure in male and female fetuses may arise and spread. Eventually we may expect complete sex-dependence to characterize the expression of genes that influence prenatal hormonal levels. That is, male fetuses will not experience high estrogen, and female fetuses will not experience high testosterone.

The distribution of the 2D:4D ratio shows a high degree of overlap between males and females. This suggests that sex-dependent expression is incomplete. Why is this so? Sex limitation is a complex adaptation, involving the evolution of sex-specific regulatory sequences (Rice 1996a). It will therefore evolve slowly. However, other things being equal, it will eventually evolve. So do we simply need more time or are there other factors operating here? One possibility is the occurrence of cycles of intragenomic conflict. Males, because they produce low-cost sperm, are able to fertilize many eggs. Females, because they produce high-cost ova and invest energy in pregnancy and lactation, are limited to smaller numbers of offspring. In populations with polygyny or frequent extra-pair copulations, the variance of male reproductive success is high. That is, a small proportion of successful males may fertilize a high proportion of eggs. When strict monogamy is practiced by most females, the variance in male reproductive success is similar to that of females. Now polygyny or extra-pair copulation may be a successful female strategy if there is substantial heritable variance in male fitness. In such a breeding system many females could mate with a few males who possessed "good genes." If there is little additive genetic variance in male fitness, female monogamy would be favored.

Suppose there are two loci controlling in utero hormonal exposure, one influencing testosterone levels, the other estrogen. A mutation arises at the testosterone locus of a male that increases in utero production of androgen. He has high testosterone levels and sperm counts, and these traits are passed on to his sons. However, because sex dependence is incomplete, his daughters have reduced fertility. The existence of a high-fitness male or small numbers of such males increases the variance in male fitness and favors a polygynous or EPC strategy in females. The high-testosterone mutation will spread, and with it the frequency of polygyny or EPCs will increase. However, as the mutation becomes common, the variance in male fitness reduces, and females may be expected to switch to increasing frequencies of monogamy. Now conditions favor the spread of a mutation at the estrogen locus that increases in utero estrogen exposure. Cycles of high prenatal testosterone and high prenatal estrogen will occur. This is interlocus coevolution of sexually antagonistic genes. Such coevolution has the characteristics of the Red Queen process (Rice and Holland 1997). That is, like the Red Queen in *Through the Looking Glass* who runs fast to merely stay in one place, change is succeeded by change without any overall directional effect. Sexually antagonistic genes should affect fertility and, because of population cycles, may be at different frequencies in different populations. Is there any evidence that 2D:4D correlates with reproductive success and that human populations differ in their mean 2D:4D ratios?

Low 2D:4D ratios are associated with high sperm counts and testosterone levels in men. Therefore 2D:4D may correlate negatively with male reproductive success. High 2D:4D ratios are associated with high estrogen and luteinizing hormones in women. Therefore, 2D:4D may correlate positively with fertility in women.

2D:4D and Reproductive Success

Associations between 2D:4D ratio and offspring number in samples drawn from a number of human populations have been reported by Manning, Barley et al. (2000) and Henzi, Manning, Venkataramana and Singh (manuscript). I will now consider these data sample by sample.

England

The participants were 411 men and women from the Merseyside area. The sample consisted of 190 men and 221 women of 30 years and over. Reproductive success is at least in part dependent on the fertility of one's partner. Therefore, couples ($n = 90$) were recruited. The mean number of offspring per participant was low (1.77 ± 1.37 children).

Family size is dependent on age. I report associations with the effect of age removed. One-tailed p values are given for negative relationships between 2D:4D and numbers of children in men and for positive relationships for women. For brevity the associations are given for the right hand only. As expected in English men, there was a negative relationship between 2D:4D and number of children ($b = -5.50$, $t = 2.01$, $p = 0.04$). In women a positive association between 2D:4D and fecundity was found ($b = 6.11$, $t = 2.65$, $p = 0.009$).

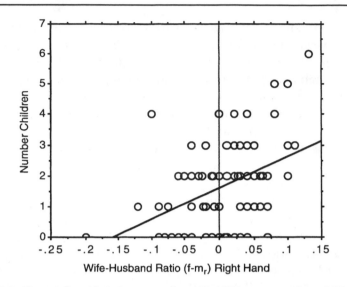

Figure 4.1. The relationship between numbers of children per couple and 2D:4D ratio of females minus 2D:4D ratio of their partner $(f - m_r)$. Women with high 2D:4D may be very fertile, while men with low 2D:4D may also be very fertile. In support of this positive values of $f - m_r$ are associated with high offspring number and negative values with low offspring number ($b = 10.16$, $t = 4.15$, $p = 0.0001$).

The couples had a mean duration of relationship of 27 ± 11.92 years. Low 2D:4D is likely to be associated with high male fertility, and high 2D:4D with high female fertility. Therefore, a composite measure of fertility per couple ($f - m_r$ = female 2D:4D − male 2D:4D) was calculated. It was found that $f - m_r$ was strongly and positively associated with number of children (see figure 4.1).

Germany

There were 238 participants of whom 205 subjects (109 men and 96 women) were aged 30 years and over. Subjects were recruited from tango studios in Bielefield, Hannover, Hamburg, and Kassel, and from staff in the Universities of Kiel, Kassel, and Hannover. The mean number of offspring per subject was small (2.29 ± 1.65 children). There was a negative relationship between male 2D:4D ratio and number of children that was not significant ($b = -1.74$, $t = 0.57$, $p = 0.29$). In women there was a significant positive relationship ($b = 6.91$, $t = 2.38$, $p = 0.01$).

Spain

A total of 98 participants (44 men and 54 women) were recruited from the Granada area of Spain. The mean number of children per subject was small (2.29 ± 1.65). Marital status was a predictor of fertility in this sample (8 subjects were unmarried and were also nulliparous). The effect of duration of marriage on number of offspring was therefore removed. There was a significant negative relationship between male 2D:4D and number of children ($b = -9.74$, $t = 2.28$, $p = 0.02$) and a positive nonsignificant relationship between 2D:4D and offspring number in women ($b = 6.93$, $t = 1.51$, $p = 0.07$).

Hungary

The subjects were recruited from southern Hungary, in and around the city of Pecs. The participants were drawn from a wide range of socio-economic backgrounds from urban and rural areas. Measurements were made in the University of Pecs, in health clinics, and in the company of health visitors in rural homes. There were 96 participants over the age of 30. The sample contained two groups, ethnic Hungarians (12 men and 39 women) and Hungarian Gypsies (15 men and 30 women). In cases of doubt ethnicity was confirmed by the health visitor or district nurse.

There were significant differences in the mean number of offspring per subject in the ethnic Hungarian and Gypsy sample (ethnic Hungarians 2.41 ± 1.15 children; Gypsies 3.48 ± 1.75 children, $t = 3.56$, $p = 0.0006$). The effects of ethnicity and of age were therefore removed. There was a negative nonsignificant relationship between male 2D:4D and numbers of children ($b = -3.87$, $t = 0.45$, $p = 0.24$) and a significant positive relationship in females ($b = 11.45$, $t = 2.27$, $p = 0.02$).

Poland

Subjects were recruited from the Poznan area of Poland. There were 210 participants over the age of 30, 107 men and 103 women. The mean number of children per participant was small (2.14 ± 1.19). The effect of age on number of children was removed. In contrast to the general trend there was a positive relationship between 2D:4D and number of children in men and a negative association in women. However, neither of the associations were significant (men, $b = 3.55$, $t = 0.87$, $p = 0.38$; women, $b = -4.93$, $t = 0.21$, $p = 0.23$).

Jamaica

The subjects were recruited from Southfield in the parish of St. Elizabeth. This is a rural area in the south of the island. The participants were 60 women who were over the age of 30 and who had at least one child attending primary school. Nulliparous women were not represented in the sample. The mean number of children was 2.93 ± 1.58, but this may be slightly above average for the area as women with no children were not included in the sample. The effect of age on number of children was removed. As with most of the female samples there was a positive relationship between 2D:4D and number of children, but this was not significant ($b = 6.88, t = 1.08, p = 0.15$).

India

The participants were recruited from two tribal groups: the Yanadi and Sugali of southern India. All measurements were made by Palla Venkataramana. There were 160 subjects (106 Yanadi and 54 Sugali) made up of 80 men and 80 women. This sample had a mean age (23.03 ± 3.36 years) lower than that of the other samples. Perhaps as a consequence the mean number of children was also low (1.75 ± 3.36 offspring). After the effects of age and ethnicity were removed, men had a nonsignificant negative relationship between 2D:4D and number of offspring ($b = -3.33, t = 0.98, p = 0.15$). Women showed a positive relationship between 2D:4D and family size that was close to formal significance ($b = 4.73, t = 1.59, p = 0.058$).

South Africa

The participants were Zulus recruited from rural areas of Natal. There were 138 subjects with 66 men and 72 women. All subjects were over age 30, and family size was also high (8.86 ± 3.96 children). The effect of age was removed from the data. In men there was a significant negative relationship between 2D:4D ratio and number of children ($b = -29.72, t = 1.70, p = 0.04$). In contrast to most of the other samples, there was a negative association between 2D:4D ratio and offspring number in women, but this was not significant ($b = -28.11, t = 1.82, p = 0.07$).

The Total Sample

An overall impression of these data is that the relationships between 2D:4D ratio and offspring number are negative in males and positive in females. We have seven samples of males and eight of females. There were six male samples showing negative relationships and one showing a positive association. Three of these samples (English, Spanish, and South African) showed significant negative associations. In the female sample there were six positive relationships between 2D:4D and family size in a total of eight samples. Three of these (English, German, and Hungarian) showed significant positive relationships. Adjustment for multiple tests is obviously necessary. Strict application of the Bonferroni correction severely reduces the power of tests (Wright 1992). Such loss of power can be reduced by choosing a 10% level of significance as suggested by Wright (1992) and Chandler (1995). Correcting within sex left significant relationships in females in the English ($p = 0.03$) and German ($p = 0.07$) samples. I think we are left with an impression of weak but nevertheless real relationships between 2D:4D and number of children, and these relationships are independent of age. Correction for multiple tests indicates that the positive relationship between female 2D:4D and family size is stronger than the negative male association. However, we have not yet corrected for population effects.

It may be inappropriate to simply pool these data without correcting for those populations with extremes of 2D:4D and offspring number. Genes that are sexually antagonistic in their effects may differ in frequency in different populations at different times with changes in the mating system, frequency of extra-pair copulations, et cetera. Furthermore, in pooled samples differences between populations in 2D:4D ratio and mean offspring number may result in strong but misleading associations. Pooling all these data results in significant negative relationships between 2D:4D and offspring number in both males and females; i.e., low 2D:4D individuals have more offspring than high 2D:4D participants (see figure 4.2). However, the Zulu sample has both low 2D:4D ratios and high numbers of children, and this sample may be having a disproportionate effect on the direction of the relationships. It is therefore necessary to control for population effects in addition to age. A simultaneous multiple regression analysis was performed with 2D:4D ratio, age, and population (dummy coded in no particular order as follows: England = 1, Germany = 2, Spain = 3, Hungary = 4 for ethnic Hungarians and 5 for Gypsies, Poland = 6, Jamaica = 7, India = 8 [Yanadi] and 9 [Sugali], and South Africa = 10) as independent variables and number of children as the independent variable. In males the independent variables in the analysis accounted for 40% of the variance in offspring number ($F = 131.53$, $p = 0.0001$). The 2D:4D ratio remained significantly and negatively related to number of children ($b = -10.90$, $t = 3.81$, $p = 0.0002$), while age ($b = 0.06$, $t = 8.43$, $p = 0.0001$) and population ($b = 0.58$, $t = 17.27$, $p = 0.0001$) were also associated with offspring number. In females the independent variables in the analysis accounted for 29% of the variance of offspring number ($F = 111.05$, $p = 0.0001$). The 2D:4D ratio was now positively but not significantly related to offspring number ($b = 0.97$, $t = 0.52$, $p = 0.60$), while age ($b = 0.04$, $t = 8.44$, $p = 0.0001$) and population ($b = 0.40$, $t = 16.55$, $p - 0.0001$) were significantly associated with offspring number.

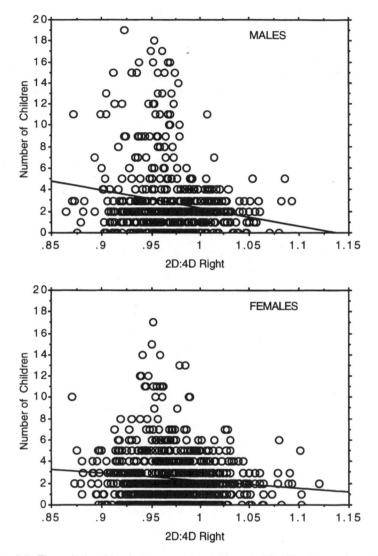

Figure 4.2. The relationships between male and female 2D:4D ratios and number of offspring in 629 men and 826 women recruited from 10 populations. There was a negative relationship between male 2D:4D ratio and number of offspring ($b = -16.79$, $F = 22.01$, $p = 0.0001$); i.e., low-ratio men had more children, which remained significant after the effects of age and population were removed. In females there was a negative relationship ($b = -6.57$, $F = 10.18$, $p = 0.002$) but this became positive and nonsignificant when age and population effects were removed.

Conclusions

Overall, the data support the position that 2D:4D ratio is a predictor of reproductive success independent of both age and population effects. Males with low values of 2D:4D have greatest reproductive success, while females with high 2D:4D are most fecund. Because age and population effects have been removed, the relationships probably reflect lifetime reproductive success and appear to be widespread in human populations. The associations are weak, and this is understandable because many factors affect the number of children produced per individual. Nevertheless, the fact that we can see these relationships at all suggests that the 2D:4D ratio is a strong predictor of individual fertility.

CHAPTER 5

Hand Preference, Verbal Fluency, Autism, and Depression

Exposure to testosterone in utero may be essential to ensure high male fertility. However, testosterone can also have negative effects on the fetus, and these need to be understood before we can appreciate the full range of selective pressures operating on genes for prenatal testosterone production. In this chapter I discuss evidence that indicates damage to the nervous system, and particularly to the brain, may result from high prenatal exposure to testosterone. Of course, this does not always occur in a striking way. Many individuals may experience high testosterone and escape serious impairment. However, it seems likely that high fetal testosterone will leave effects that may range in severity from profoundly deleterious to subtle but significant changes in brain function. For example, testosterone could precipitate autism, a serious childhood condition that includes delayed or absent language among its symptoms. The frequency of births of children with autism is quite rare, but compromised abilities in aspects of language such as verbal fluency are not. Autism may well result in a profound reduction in fitness. Reductions in verbal fluency could, for example, compromise courtship and have subtle but overall negative effects on mate choice. It is in the context of deleterious effects of prenatal testosterone that I discuss hand preference, verbal fluency, autism, and depression. Note that it is not clear that preference for the left hand is a deleterious trait in itself, or even a marker for lowered phenotypic quality. I include it here because it sits equally uncomfortably with the advantageous traits associated with prenatal testosterone, e.g., enhanced visual-spatial perception and musical and sporting abilities. These latter traits will be dealt with in chapters 8 and 9.

Testosterone and the Brain

Prenatal testosterone has been implicated in the development of a number of extragenital organ systems including the central nervous system (Bardin and Caterall 1981; McEwen 1981; MacLusky and Naftolin 1981). Androgens are probably the most important gonadal hormones for the organization of the brain. Testosterone is transformed into estradiol within the brain, and it is estradiol that is the activating factor in maturation and differentiation. Receptors for estradiol are found in the fetal cortex but not in the brains of adults. Aromatase is the enzyme that turns testosterone into estradiol. Receptors for androgen and many neurons producing aromatase have been found in the fetal hypothalamus. These neurons show higher estradiol formation in males compared to females (Hutchison et al. 1997). In three influential but controversial papers Geschwind and Galaburda (1985a, 1985b, 1985c) have set out evidence for the processes that lead to an asymmetric nervous system. These papers were followed two years later by a book in which most of the points made in the 1985 papers were reiterated (Geschwind and Galaburda 1987). Central to their thesis was the effect of prenatal testosterone on the development of left-handedness and developmental disorders such as autism, dyslexia, migraine, and stuttering, and abilities such as visual-spatial judgment, music, and mathematics. In addition they postulated in utero testosterone influenced other systems such as the skin and skeleton and had a depressive effect on the immune system.

Geschwind and Galaburda suggested that prenatal testosterone tends to retard the growth of certain areas of the left hemisphere while enhancing the growth of comparable areas in the right hemisphere. Language skills will therefore be negatively affected while hand preference will tend to be shifted toward the left. On the positive side the fetus that produces high testosterone concentrations may enjoy enhanced right hemisphere skills such as visual-spatial processing and mathematical and musical abilities. The Geschwind-Galaburda model is controversial. Predicted associations between lateralized hand performance and immune disorders, autism, and dyslexia have not always been supported by follow-up studies (Bryden et al. 1994; Gilger et al. 1992; Gilger et al. 1992). A more powerful test of the model would be to relate these traits to prenatal testosterone concentrations. It is not possible to do this directly, but if 2D:4D is a correlate of prenatal testosterone its pattern of expression may be that predicted by Geschwind and Galaburda. In this chapter I examine evidence for the association between low 2D:4D ratios and a shift toward left-hand preference, compromised verbal fluency, an elevated risk of autism, and a tendency (not predicted by Geschwind and Galaburda) toward depression.

Left-Lateralized Hand Performance

This work was carried out on 285 rural Jamaican children (156 boys and 129 girls) aged 5 to 11 years (Manning, Trivers et al. 2000) and was part of a long-term study, the Jamaican Symmetry Project (for an introduction to the study, see Trivers et al. 1999). Hand performance was measured with an Annett peg-moving task. A pegboard with two rows of 10 pegs was used. The subjects moved the pegs from one row to an empty row situated about 13 centimeters in front. There were 10 trials, 5 for each hand, and mean times for the right and left hands were calculated. Lateralized hand performance (LHP) was calculated by dividing the right-hand time by the left-hand time. Therefore, low LHP indicated a right-hand advantage for speed and a high LHP a left-hand advantage. The measures of LHP were made in January 1996 on 250 participants selected at random from our study population. They had a mean LHP of 0.88 ± 0.07; that is, most participants had a faster right-hand performance than left. As expected boys had a higher tendency toward left-lateralized performance than girls (LHP: boys 0.88 ± 0.07, girls 0.87 ± 0.08), but this fell just short of significance ($t = 1.92, p = 0.055$).

The 2D:4D ratio was measured from two sources. Photocopies were made of the right and left hands of 152 children (78 boys and 74 girls) in June 1998. X-rays were also taken from the dorsal surface of the right and left hands of 244 children (135 boys and 109 girls) in January 1996. The photocopies were made 2.5 years after the X-rays. Nevertheless, in the 135 children for whom there were both X-rays and photocopies, there was a significant relationship between the 2D:4D ratios calculated from the two different sources (right hand $r = 0.46, p = 0.0001$; left hand $r = 0.47$, $p = 0.0001$). This suggests that the ratio is stable over time.

In the photocopied sample there was a significant negative relationship in boys and girls between 2D:4D ratio of the right hand but not the left. High LHP was associated with low 2D:4D ratio and the association was significant for the right hand (see figure 5.1). This result was consistent with relationships between low 2D:4D, high prenatal testosterone, and left-hand preference. There were the same general trends in the X-ray sample. However, the right-hand 2D:4D ratio was significantly related to LHP in boys only ($b = -0.56, F = 5.42, p = 0.01$ one-tailed adjusted for multiple tests $p = 0.04$).

Jamaicans have low 2D:4D ratios, and presumably high intrauterine concentrations of testosterone are common for males and females. In such populations a greater right-hand sensitivity to androgens compared to the left hand may lead to markedly negative values of D_{r-l} being associated with very high prenatal testosterone (see chapter 1). It was found that D_{r-l} was negatively correlated with an increasing speed of use of the left hand compared to right hand in boys and girls measured from photocopies and from X-rays (see figure 5.2).

It appears from these results that low 2D:4D ratios, particularly low right-hand 2D:4D ratios relative to left hand, are associated with left-lateralized preference. As there is evidence for an association between

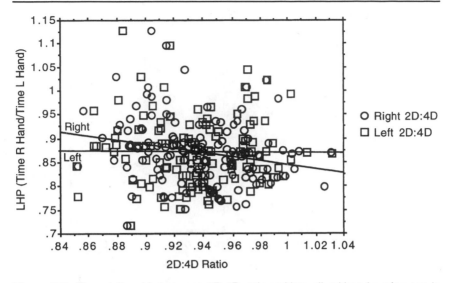

Figure 5.1. The relationship between 2D:4D ratio and lateralized hand preference in 130 Jamaican children. Measurements were made from photocopies of the hand. High LHP indicates a fast left-hand performance. Low 2D:4D in the right hand is correlated with high LHP (right hand, $b = -0.36$, $F = 4.51$, $p = 0.01$ one-tailed test, Bonferroni adjusted $p = 0.02$; left hand $b = -0.02$, $F = 0.02$, $p = 0.90$).

low 2D:4D ratios and high in utero testosterone, I conclude that these data support an association between prenatal testosterone and left-hand preference.

Verbal Fluency

Verbal fluency tasks show reliable sex differences with women usually out-performing men (McGlone 1986; Halpern 1992). The left frontal and cortical lobes are believed to be particularly responsible for this activity (Lezak 1983). Manning and Mather Hillon (manuscript) have used tests of semantically and phonologically based fluency to examine associations with 2D:4D ratio in a sample of 100 men and 100 women.

Phonologically based fluency was tested by the FAS test. Subjects were asked to list as many words as possible beginning with the letters *F, A,* or *S* in three 90-second sessions. Semantically based verbal fluency was tested using the Varley test (Varley 1995). Subjects were asked to list as many words as possible in three 90-second sessions belonging to the categories "animals," "politicians," and "singers/musicians." In men there were positive associations between mean 2D:4D ratio and fluency for both tests, and the relationship between 2D:4D and semantically based verbal fluency was

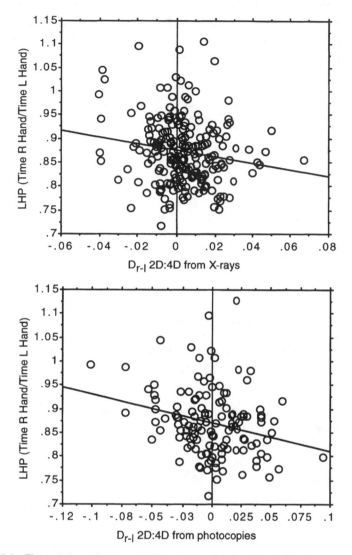

Figure 5.2. The relationship between D_{r-l} (right 2D:4D minus left 2D:4D) and lateralized hand preference in Jamaican children. The 2D:4D ratio was measured from photocopies ($n = 131$) and X-rays ($n = 214$). High LHP indicates a fast left-hand performance relative to the right hand. Negative values (i.e., malelike) of D_{r-l} are associated with high LHP; i.e., subjects with low right 2D:4D compared to their left 2D:4D ratio have an increased left-hand preference (photocopies $b = -0.60$, $F = 8.64$, $p = 0.004$, adjusted for multiple tests $p = 0.008$; X-rays $b = -0.68$, $F = 5.51$, $p = 0.02$).

significant (see figure 5.3). Although age may be related to verbal fluency, the results of a multiple regression test showed both age (negatively) and 2D:4D (positively) were independently related to the Varley test results for males (age $b = -0.14$, $t = 2.75$, $p = 0.007$; mean 2D:4D $b = 65.41$, $t = 3.48$, $p = 0.008$). The situation in the female sample was similar, with positive

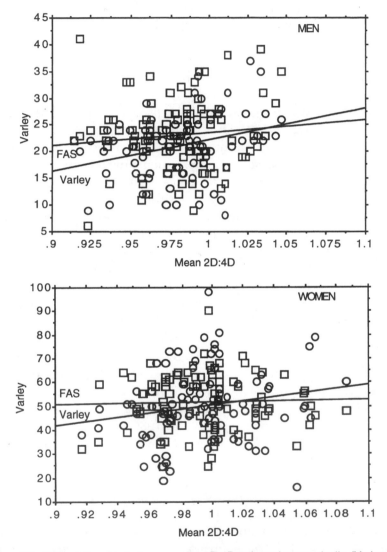

Figure 5.3. The relationship between mean 2D:4D ratio and semantically (Varley test, men $b = 58.51$, $F = 9.22$, $p = 0.003$, adjusted for multiple tests $p = 0.01$; women $b = 86.56$, $F = 3.59$, $p = 0.06$) and phonologically (FAS test, men $b = 23.84$, $F = 1.04$, $p = 0.31$; women $b = 9.80$, $F = 0.07$, $p = 0.79$) based fluency in 100 men and 100 women. Men with low 2D:4D ratio have reduced semantically based fluency.

associations between 2D:4D and fluency. The strongest relationship was again with the Varley test, but neither association was significant. There was also the suggestion in these data that men with low 2D:4D in the right hand relative to the left had lower fluency, but this was not significant (D_{r-l}; FAS $b = 16.81$, $F = 1.08$, $p = 0.30$; Varley $b = 24.26$, $F = 3.1$, $p = 0.08$).

I conclude that the negative relationship between 2D:4D and the Varley test supports the hypothesis that high prenatal testosterone compromises verbal fluency.

Autism

Autism is the most severe of the childhood psychiatric disorders (American Psychiatric Association 1994). It is strongly heritable (Bailey et al. 1995) and is diagnosed on the basis of deficits in social development, communication, and imagination (i.e., impairments in the development of a theory of mind). Characteristically, there is a history of language delay. However, a subgroup of people with autism or Asperger Syndrome (AS) share the social and communicative symptoms of autism but have no history of language delay (for a general treatment of autism, see Frith 1989; Baron-Cohen and Bolton 1993).

Children with autism are often unresponsive to people, treat individuals as inanimate objects, show lack of eye contact, disregard cultural norms, show attention to nonsocial aspects of people, and show a lack of awareness of the feelings of others. The inability to judge other people's thoughts is a particularly crucial trait in autism. Children with autism have a form of "mindblindness" (Baron-Cohen 1995) that prevents them from developing a concept or theory of mind. Predicting people's actions and understanding deception are particularly difficult for children with autism.

The pattern of autism is one which suggests an association with testosterone (Geschwind and Galaburda 1985a, 1985b, 1985c). There are more boys with autism than girls. The male to female sex ratio is 4:1 across the full IQ range (Rutter 1978), rising to 9:1 among children with AS (Wing 1981). In addition some children with autism have "islets" of ability that may be the result of testosterone-driven enhancement of the right hemisphere. The abilities include music, drawing, finding shapes within patterns, and calendar calculation (Baron-Cohen and Bolton 1993). Males often score higher than females in tasks that test visual, spatial, and mathematical skills (Halpern 1992; Voyer 1996). The incidence of autism is elevated over population norms in relatives of students of mathematics, physics, and engineering, and fathers and grandfathers of children with autism have an increased probability of being engineers (Baron-Cohen et al. 1997). This pattern of the expression of autism has led to the development of the "extreme male brain theory of autism" (Baron-Cohen and Hammer 1997).

Models that invoke poor parenting (psychogenic theory; see Bettelheim 1967) as a cause of autism appear to be unsupported by any persuasive data. In contrast the biological theory enjoys substantial empirical support. The biological theory concerns the effect on the developing brain of several factors, e.g., genes, testosterone, complications during pregnancy, or viral infections. The evidence for genetic effects is compelling. Within families with a child with autism, there is about a 2 or 3% probability of a brother or sister with the condition. This compares to a population norm of 1 in 1,000 births. Lesser learning problems of similar type to autism present with increased frequency in first-degree relatives (Bolton et al. 1994; Baron-Cohen and Hammer 1997). Studies of autism in monozygotic and dizygotic twins have shown higher concordance rates in the former compared to the latter (Bailey et al. 1995).

Developmental instability may arise from such factors as harmful mutations and the effects of prenatal testosterone. Early fetal maldevelopment is associated with minor physical anomalies (MPAs). Autistic children have been shown to have elevated levels of MPAs, e.g., fused, curved, and crooked digits and toes, compared to their siblings and controls (Campbell et al. 1978; Links et al. 1980; Links 1980; Gualtieri et al. 1982; Rodier et al. 1997) and perturbations in fingerprint patterns compared to controls (Walker 1976; Arrieta et al. 1993). In addition to MPAs there are a number of congenital anomaly syndromes that have been associated with an increased incidence of autism (Baron-Cohen and Bolton 1993). At least some of these involve perturbations in formation of the digits (Cornelia de Lange syndrome—small hands and feet; Biedle-Bardet syndrome—extra digits) or in the formation of the heart (Noonan syndrome, William's syndrome), which may suggest an involvement with prenatal testosterone (see chapter 6). Developmental instability may be correlated with cellular malfunction in addition to phenodeviance. A number of studies have suggested a disturbance in ATP production in subjects with autism. Children with autism may have elevated levels of serum lactate (Coleman and Blass 1985), evidence of impaired flurodeoxyglucose uptake (Fchifter 1994), increased instability of brain membranes with reduced high-energy phosphate levels (Minshew et al. 1993), and mitochondrial dysfunction (Lombard 1998).

Prenatal testosterone may be one important causative factor in this constellation of brain dysfunction and brain enhancement. The working hypothesis is therefore that (a) children with autism will have lower 2D:4D ratios than non-autistic controls; (b) children with AS will have higher

2D:4D ratios than children with autism; (c) fathers and mothers of children with autism will have lower 2D:4D ratios than those of controls; and (d) there will be evidence of heritability of 2D:4D ratios within families with children with autism.

Manning, Baron-Cohen et al. (2001) examined these predictions. The sample included 72 children with autism (23 subjects with AS), 34 unaffected siblings, 88 fathers, 88 mothers, and their controls matched for sex and age. Children with autism had lower mean 2D:4D ratios than controls and lower mean 2D:4D than AS children; siblings of children with autism had lower mean 2D:4D ratios than controls; mothers had lower mean 2D:4D ratios than controls; and fathers also had lower mean 2D:4D ratios than controls (see figure 5.4).

Autism is strongly heritable. If there is genetically influenced variance in the severity of autism then we would expect the same for mean 2D:4D

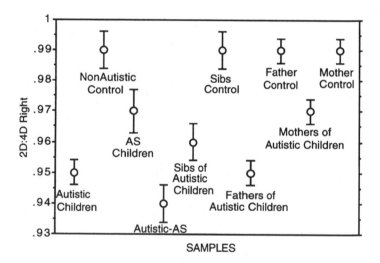

Figure 5.4. Means and standard error bars for ten right-hand 2D:4D ratios from autistic children and controls, Asperger's Syndrome children and controls, autistic children with AS children removed, siblings of autistic children and controls, fathers of autistic children and controls, and mothers of autistic children and controls. In comparison with controls mean 2D:4D ratios were significantly lower in samples drawn from children with autism (autistic, 0.95 ± 0.004SE, controls 0.99 ± 0.006SE, paired t test used throughout, $t = 5.21$, $p = 0.0001$, Bonferroni corrected $p = 0.0004$), AS children (autistic, 0.94 ± 0.006SE, AS, 0.97 ± 0.007SE, $t = 3.37$, $p = 0.001$, Bonferonni corrected $p = 0.001$), their siblings (siblings 0.96 ± 0.006SE, controls 0.99 ± 0.004SE, $t = 5.27$, $p = 0.0001$, Bonferroni corrected $p = 0.0003$), fathers (fathers, 0.95 ± 0.004SE, controls 0.99 ± 0.004SE, $t = 6.01$, $p = 0.0001$, Bonferroni corrected $p = 0.0003$), and mothers (mothers 0.97 ± 0.004, controls 0.99 ± 0.004, $t = 3.72$, $p = 0.0001$, Bonferroni corrected $p = 0.003$).

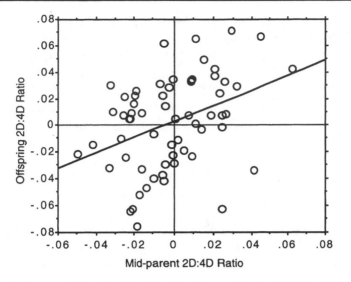

Figure 5.5. A regression of offspring 2D:4D ratio on mid-parent 2D:4D ratio. The heritability is quite high (heritability $h^2 = 0.58 \pm 0.19$ standard error). Calculated from families with autistic children.

ratio. Accordingly, a regression of the mean 2D:4D of children with autism (including children with AS) on mid-parent 2D:4D (i.e., mean parental 2D:4D) gave a significant heritability of 0.58 (see figure 5.5). It must be emphasized that this does not mean that parents with low 2D:4D ratios will have children with autism. Rather, it suggests that low parental 2D:4D ratios are associated with an increased chance of autism in the children. Other factors such as developmental instability, viral infections, and trauma during pregnancy or at birth may all conspire to increase the probability of autism. One way forward in this is to investigate further correlates of parental testosterone levels. In addition to 2D:4D ratios, we may find that the waist:hip ratio of mothers is associated with the autistic phenotype of their children. High waist:hip ratio is found in women with high serum concentrations of testosterone (Evans et al. 1983). In addition, the waist:hip ratio of women is negatively associated with their 2D:4D ratio and the waist:hip ratio of mothers is negatively correlated with the 2D:4D ratio of their children (Manning et al. 1999). High maternal and paternal waist:hip ratio may be a further predictor of autism in children.

Depression

Depression is a mood disturbance. Symptoms include loss of appetite, insomnia, early morning awakening, thoughts of suicide, crying, memory problems, worrying, hypochondria, and irritability. Women tend to report higher rates and more intensity of depression than men. Some have felt that this sex difference in rates and intensity of depression may result from low testosterone in women and in some men. Therefore, a number of studies have explored the hypothesis that lowered testosterone levels are associated with depression, and that testosterone concentration rises on recovery (Vogel et al. 1978; Levitt and Joffe 1988; Davies et al. 1992; Steiger et al. 1993). The results from these studies have been equivocal, and there is no consensus as to the effects of testosterone on the probability of presentation of depression or on its progression. Men tend to feel shame at reporting depression, and sex-dependent rates of reported depression may be unreliable. Depression and poor impulse control are considered common precursors of suicide (Gross-Isseroff et al. 1990). Females are more likely to attempt suicide than males, in a ratio of between 2:1 to 8:1, but males are more likely to be successful, in a ratio of about 4:1 to 5:1 (Holden 1986). It is not known whether the high rates of male suicide reflect a tendency in men to use instantaneously lethal methods such as shooting or hanging, or that very intense and often unreported depression is more common in males compared to females. Depression and poor impulse control may be influenced by genes and brain chemistry, and suicide may show an inherited predisposition (Gross-Isseroff et al. 1990). We are concerned here with the prenatal effects of testosterone. Magnetic resonance imaging (MRI) findings in patients with depression confirm the existence of higher frequency of various brain lesions compared to controls (see Videbech 1997 for a meta-analysis of MRI studies on patients with affective disorders). If high concentrations of in utero testosterone are associated with autism, dyslexia, stammering, and migraine in males, and these conditions can themselves be associated with brain lesions (see Baron-Cohen and Bolton 1993 for autism), then it may be that the etiology of male depression could also be associated with prenatal testosterone.

Martin et al. (1999) have considered the relationship between reported depression scores and digit length in men and women. The participants were 102 Liverpool residents (52 men and 50 women). Recruitment was from north Liverpool and the catchment area included a wide range of socioeconomic groups. Volunteers were recruited from a variety of sources. An attempt was made to include subjects who had high depression scores, and some participants were from clinical sources. This probably increased the variance in the depression scores, so that they were not necessarily representative of population norms.

Depression was measured using the Beck Depression Inventory (BDI). The BDI is a 21-item questionnaire designed to measure the severity of depression in adolescents and adults (Beck and Steer 1984). It includes questions on such feelings as sadness, guilt, disappointment, irritation, indecision, and physical problems including insomnia, tiredness, poor appetite, weight loss, and low sex drive. Although it was not originally designed as a diagnostic instrument, the BDI has been used to detect depression in normal populations and in psychiatric patients (Steer et al. 1985). Digit length was measured for the 2nd to 5th digits inclusively.

The BDI scores had a median of 7 and varied from 0 to 49. The distribution was strongly skewed toward low BDI scores. As expected, males had lower median BDI scores than females (males, median 5, range 0 to 24; females, median 8, range 0 to 49) and this gender difference was significant (log $[1 + x]$ transformed scores, $t = 2.60$, $p = 0.01$). There was no significant relationship between the BDI and age, height, or weight for the total sample or for either sex; for example, for men: age $b = -0.005$, $p = 0.30$; height $b = -0.06$, $p = 0.84$; weight $b = 0.002$, $p = 0.29$.

Digit length proved to be significantly and positively related to BDI scores in men but not women. That is, men with long fingers tended to report more intense depression than men with short fingers. These relationships were present for absolute digit length and digit length corrected for height, although the associations were stronger for the latter (see table 5.1 and figure 5.6 for association between BDI and right 4D/height). In this case 4th digit length divided by height (m²) did not show stronger associations with the index trait (BDI) than 4th digit length divided by height (m) alone.

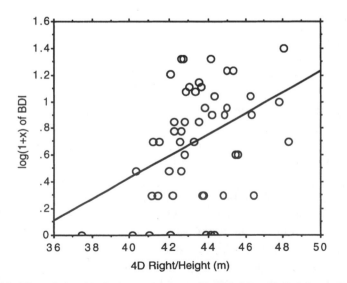

Figure 5.6. The relationship between the mean length of the 4th digit (mm) divided by height (meters) and the Beck Depression Index (BDI) in 52 men. Subjects with long 4th digits corrected for height reported more intense depression scores.

Table 5.1. Relationships between digit length corrected for height and Beck Depression Scores

Trait	Adjusted values (beta)	F	p
Men: Right Hand			
2nd Digit	62.16	4.89	0.03 (0.045)
3rd Digit	62.35	5.16	0.03 (0.045)
4th Digit	79.65	8.64	0.005 (0.02)
5th Digit	70.86	6.72	0.01 (0.03)
Men: Left Hand			
2nd Digit	71.71	6.41	0.01 (0.03)
3rd Digit	70.08	7.11	0.01 (0.03)
4th Digit	82.75	10.72	0.002 (0.01)
5th Digit	57.43	3.97	0.052 (0.052)
Women: Right Hand			
2nd Digit	0.01	0.52	0.47
3rd Digit	0.002	0.02	0.89
4th Digit	0.01	0.35	0.55
5th Digit	0.005	0.12	0.73
Women: Left Hand			
2nd Digit	0.01	0.35	0.55
3rd Digit	0.002	0.01	0.91
4th Digit	0.01	0.76	0.39
5th Digit	0.01	0.55	0.46

The relationship between 2D:4D ratio and log $(1 + x)$ BDI was a negative one in men; i.e., men with low 2D:4D reported high depression scores. However, this association was not significant (right hand $b = -38.91$, $F = 1.72$, $p = 0.20$; left hand $b = -53.08$, $F = 3.22$, $p = 0.08$). It is possible that this is, in fact, a real relationship and it should be investigated further. In women there was no relationship between 2D:4D ratio and log $(1 + x)$ BDI (mean 2D:4D $b = -0.09$, $F = 0.004$, $p = 0.95$). There were no significant associations between D_{r-l} and depression in men ($b = 40.26$, $F = 0.57$, $p = 0.45$) or women ($b = 112.47$, $F = 1.80$, $p = 0.19$).

These data indicate that a likely marker for prenatal testosterone, the length of the 4th digit corrected for height, is positively correlated with depression in men. High levels of fetal testosterone may be an important causative factor in male depression. Although depression in females is a major problem and one that should not be minimized, the etiology of male and female affective disorders may be different.

Conclusions

I have discussed the relationships between 2D:4D ratio and three delete-rious traits: compromised verbal fluency, autism, and depression. There are likely to be many more that are at least partly dependent on fetal tes-tosterone. For example, perturbations in digit dermatoglyphics formed before 19 weeks of gestation have been reported to be correlated with adult testosterone concentrations (Jamison et al. 1993) and to the inci-dence of schizophrenia (Markow and Wandler 1986). The 2D:4D ratio could prove useful in providing evidence that implicates prenatal testos-terone in the etiology of sex-dependent traits and behaviors such as autism, dyslexia, difficulties in language acquisition, stammering, mi-graine, schizophrenia, risk taking, and drug-related behavior. Psychopathy is one such trait that may be related to low 2D:4D ratio. Psychopaths are more often men than women, and they show manipulative, impulsive, and callous behavior. Characteristically they have no concern for the welfare of others and little guilt at the result of their antisocial behavior (Gacono 2000). Psychopaths are less physiologically reactive when exposed to un-expected stimuli such as loud sounds, are less reactive when anticipating aversive stimuli, are less affected by cues of distress, and they appear to process emotional cues in verbal information differently than non-psychopaths (Ogloff and Wong 1990; Patrick 1994; Williamson et al. 1991). Psychopaths often have extensive criminal histories, and compared to non-psychopaths they are more likely to commit crimes on discharge from prison, their crimes more often involve weapons, and those crimes are more often directed toward nonkin and toward male victims (review in Patrick and Zempolich 1998). There are two distinct views of psycho-pathy. It may be that the differences between psychopaths and non-psychopaths result from behavioral, emotional, physiological, and cognitive deficits (Patrick 1994). According to this view psychopathy is a deleterious trait. Alternatively, psychopathy could be an alternative male behavior that involves playing a "cheating" or short-term benefit strategy in mating and a risky aggressive approach to establishing social dominance (Mealey 1995; Lalumiere and Seto 1998). The predominance of males among psychopaths and their lack of empathy with others suggest the involvement of prenatal testosterone. I think it likely that high scores on measures of psychopathy will be correlated with low 2D:4D ratio.

CHAPTER 6

Birth Weight, Heart Attack, Breast Cancer, and Sex-Dependent Diseases

We have seen that the 2D:4D ratio may correlate with autism, verbal fluency, depression, and other traits associated with the function of the central nervous system (CNS). What of traits that may be sensitive to prenatal conditions such as birth weight, serious adult-onset diseases of organ systems other than the CNS including heart disease and breast cancer, susceptibility to viruses such as HIV, and susceptibility to parasitic infections, for example, onchocerciasis? In this chapter I discuss the data that link 2D:4D to birth weight, heart attack, and breast cancer. I also put forward hypotheses regarding the relationship between 2D:4D ratio and sex-dependent diseases such as cancers of the reproductive system (prostate, endometrial, and ovarian cancers), HIV/AIDS, and parasitic infections.

Sex-Dependent Disease Expression

Manning and Bundred (2000) have pointed out that any disease with a sex-dependent expression may have an etiology related to prenatal testosterone or estrogen exposure.

The rate of fetal development is sexually dimorphic. Females complete their developmental program faster than males. Halfway through their gestation they are three weeks more advanced than males; at birth the difference in the skeleton is four to six weeks of maturation. The differences are carried through to childhood, as girls reach 50% of their adult height earlier and begin puberty and cease growing earlier (Tanner 1990). On average, boys are heavier at birth than girls. This means that birth weight is dependent on some aspect of sex. Within each sex it is possible that prenatal testosterone tends to slow down the developmental program. Birth weight is probably a sensitive indicator of prenatal conditions, and low birth weight, particularly low male birth weight, has been shown to correlate with childhood and adult disease and morbidity, including heart disease (Neligan et al. 1976; Buck et al. 1989; Holst et al. 1989; Barker 1992).

Coronary heart disease is also strongly sex-dependent in its expression. The World Health Organization's MONICA (monitoring trends and determinants in cardiovascular disease) project followed trends in heart disease in 37 populations from 21 countries for 10 years. There were 166,000 coronary "events" registered in men and women between 35 and 64 years. Men outnumbered women in deaths resulting from heart disease by four to one (WHO MONICA Project 1988). The magnitude of the sex difference in mortality varies between populations. According to the British Heart Foundation (BHF), in Britain men are twice as likely to die from coronary heart disease as women (BHF 1996). However, there is a consistent excess of male deaths across human populations, and this accounts for a substantial part of the sex difference in overall mortality rates.

It may appear redundant to remark that breast cancer is strongly sex-dependent. However, men have breast tissue that is essentially similar to that of women's breasts, and a variety of benign and malignant breast conditions may affect men. Nevertheless, male breast cancer accounts for only 0.7% of all breast cancers (Gateley 1998).

HIV/AIDS is essentially a sexually transmitted disease. At the very beginning of the epidemic most AIDS patients were male homosexuals, intravenous drug users, or hemophiliacs (Goedert and Blattner 1985). However, it quickly became clear that male homosexuals were the largest group. In this sense expression of HIV/AIDS was sex-dependent. However, sub-Saharan Africa has now become the focus of the infection (Gilks 1999). Transmission in southern Africa is predominantly via heterosexual sexual activity. There may be sex and population differences in 2D:4D at play here that could explain the etiology of HIV/AIDS.

Many important parasitic diseases show a preponderance of male patients, or progression may be faster and prognosis worse in males (see Brabin and Brabin 1992). These include lymphatic filariasis (associated with lymphoedemia), onchocerciasis (leading to ocular lesions and "river" blindness), trypanosomiasis (giving rise to Chagas' disease in South America and sleeping sickness in Africa), visceral leishmaniasis (leading to kala azar), *Plasmodium* and Epstein-Barr virus (infection with the malarial parasite and this virus may trigger Burkitt's lymphoma). In addition *Plasmodium* may readily infect women who are pregnant for the first time, resulting in marked reductions in birth weight (Brabin 1991). The 2D:4D ratio could be predictive of susceptibility to such parasitic diseases.

Birth Weight

There are many factors which affect birth weight. I confine myself here to the possible effect of androgens.

Androgens, Birth Weight, and Developmental Patterns

Low birth weight, i.e., less than 2,500 g, or lower than expected birth weight for gestational age, is correlated with disease rates and mortality in childhood (Campbell 1989; Holst et al. 1989). Furthermore, it has recently become apparent that a number of cardiovascular and metabolic diseases of later life are related to low birth weight (Barker 1992). It is important to understand the factors that determine prenatal growth rates and developmental patterns. Variations in fetal size (crown to rump length, which correlates with birth weight) have been reported from studies using first-trimester ultrasound scans (Dickey and Gasser 1993; Smith et al. 1998). Therefore, quite early differences in prenatal conditions may contribute to variance in birth weight.

One possible influence on early developmental rates is exposure to testosterone. Male fetuses produce more testosterone than females. Although males are born heavier than females (on average about 150 g heavier; Tanner 1990) their developmental rate in utero is slower than that shown by females. There are numerous examples of this. One such is the age- and sex-dependent pattern of fetal mouth movements. Hepper et al. (1997) scanned 39 fetuses (20 female and 19 male) at 16, 18, and 20 weeks of gestation. Each scan lasted one hour, and the number of jaw movements (which may or may not have included tongue movements) were counted at each gestational age. Jaw movements increased with fetal age ($p = 0.001$), and at each gestational age females moved their mouths more than males (for all data $p = 0.02$).

Testosterone has been implicated in a reduction in developmental rates of the CNS leading to left-handedness, autism, dyslexia, migraine, and stuttering (Geschwind and Galaburda 1985a; Jamison et al. 1993), an early supression of the development of the thymus gland resulting in immune disorders of the gastrointestinal tract and the thyroid (Geschwind and Galaburda 1985b), and to an inhibition of fetal lung development (Klein and Neilsen 1993). It is therefore possible that within the sexes high in utero androgen concentrations correlate with low birth weight. In contrast to testosterone, high prenatal concentrations of estrogen are positively associated with birth weight (Sanderson et al. 1996). High prenatal testosterone and low estrogen are likely to be associated with low 2D:4D. A reasonable working hypothesis is that 2D:4D ratio is positively related to birth weight or correlates of birth weight.

2D:4D in Very Low Birth Weight Children

Manning, Stevenson, Bundred, and Pharoah (manuscript) have examined 2D:4D ratio and birth weight relationships in a cohort study of very low birth weight males and females. The sample consisted of 205 infants weighing less than 1,500 g, and born from 1979 to 1981 to mothers who resided at the time of the birth in the five health districts of the county of Merseyside. The obstetric and neonatal records were abstracted for birth weight and head circumference of the child. Expected birth weight was calculated. This was the mean for gestational age, and controlled for sex, parity (two categories, primiparae and multiparae), and plurality of birth (two categories, singleton and twin), using the 1985 and 1989 Scottish national data from 894,066 live births (Hutton et al. 1997). Children with a disability were excluded from the sample. Disability was defined as including cerebral palsy, hearing loss that required the use of a hearing aid or admission to a school for the deaf, a reduction of visual acuity of less than 6/12 in the better eye or a necessity for special schooling, a learning disability that required special schooling, and epilepsy. The children were examined at ages 3, 8, and 14. At 14 years ink prints of the ventral surface of the digits were obtained. Measurements were made from the ink prints of the 2nd and 4th digits of the right and left hands.

The digits were measured from the proximal crease of the second phalanx to the tip of the finger. This comprised the length of the two distal phalanges. Some digits gave ink prints with indistinct proximal creases, and these were not included in the study. There were 155 participants who had ink prints that were sufficiently clear to measure for one or both hands. In total 2D:4D ratios were calculated from 126 right hands and 143 left hands. The mean 2D:4D ratio of the right and left hands was calculated for 111 subjects. Handprints were taken from some subjects. Digits were also measured from these complete handprints (27 hands from 27 subjects). The 2D:4D ratios calculated from lengths of the two distal phalanges were compared with the finger ratios obtained from measurements of complete digits.

There was no significant difference between the 2D:4D ratios calculated from digit measures that included the complete digit and those that did not (paired t-test, $x - y = -0.02$, $t = 0.42$, $p = 0.68$). There were 57 males and 54 females with ratios that were measurable in both hands and a population mean of 0.94 ± 0.04 SD for mean 2D:4D. Males had a lower digit ratio than females (males, mean 2D:4D $= 0.93 \pm 0.04$ SD; females, mean 2D:4D $= 0.95 \pm 0.04$ SD, unpaired t-test, $t = 2.72$, $p = 0.007$). The mean 2D:4D ratios were lower than population norms (males 0.98 and females 1.00; Manning et al. 1998), and this may have arisen because the index group were all very low birth weight children.

There were no significant relationships between mean 2D:4D ratio and birth weight or gestational age (birth weight $b = 3.75$, $F = 0.49$, $p = 0.48$; gestational age $b = -10.68$, $F = 2.19$, $p = 0.14$). There was, however, a significant positive relationship between right-hand 2D:4D ratio and the ratio of birth weight to expected birth weight (BW/ExBW, $p = 0.02$; see figure 6.1). There was also a positive relationship between 2D:4D of the left hand and BW/ExBW, but this was not significant ($b = 0.32$, $F = 0.80$,

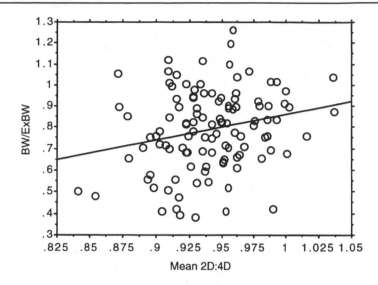

Figure 6.1. The relationship between mean 2D:4D of the right and left hands and the ratio between birth weight and expected birth weight (BW/ExBW) in 111 subjects who had very low birth weight (less than 1,500 g). Measurements of the digits were made from ink prints taken at age 14. The BW/ExBw increases with mean 2D:4D ratio ($b = 1.20$, $F = 6.07$, $p = 0.02$). That is, within this particular group of children, low 2D:4D ratio individuals are likely to have lower than expected birth weights. This may mean that prenatal testosterone tends to slow fetal development. The relationship is independent of sex.

$p = 0.37$). As expected D_{r-l} was positively related to BW/ExBW, but the association was not significant ($b = 0.40$, $F = 0.90$, $p = 0.35$).

A simultaneous multiple regression analysis with independent variables right-hand digit ratio and sex (dummy coded, males = 1, females = 2) and dependent variable BW/ExBW showed 2D:4D ratio was significantly related to BW/ExBW independent of sex (right hand 2D:4D, $b = 0.99$, $t = 2.45$, $p = 0.02$; sex, $b = 0.03$, $t = 0.84$, $p = 0.40$).

A partial correlation analysis with variables right-hand 2D:4D, birth weight, gestational age, and sex showed that 2D:4D was negatively related to gestational age ($r = -0.21$, $p = 0.04$) and independent of birth weight (2D:4D and birth weight, $r = 0.14$) or sex (2D:4D and sex, $r = 0.25$, $p = 0.01$). That is, children with low 2D:4D ratio tended to have high gestational age. It may be that mothers retain low 2D:4D ratio (i.e., high testosterone exposure) children longer in an attempt to counteract the effect that prenatal testosterone has in slowing intrauterine growth rates.

If testosterone slows down growth and development it may be that it has a negative effect on motor function. Motor impairment was tested at age eight in this cohort study. The Henderson Test for Motor Impairment was used. The test has a maximum score of 16, with higher score equal to more impairment. A total of 107 children were tested. There was a weak and nonsignificant negative association between mean 2D:4D ratio of the right and left hands and scores from the Henderson test ($b = -1.8$, $F = 0.03$, $p = 0.85$). The effect of sex was removed using a simultaneous multiple regression test. Neither 2D:4D ratio or sex were significant predictors of motor impairment (2D:4D $b = -2.54$, $t = 0.24$, $p = 0.81$; sex $b = 0.20$, $t = 0.27$, $p = 0.79$). The relationship is in the expected direction, i.e., low 2D:4D associated with more impairment, but there is little evidence here to support a role of prenatal testosterone in the etiology of motor impairment.

2D:4D and Normal Birth Weight Children

The previous data refer to very low birth weight children. What of children with birth weight within the normal range? Is low birth weight associated with low 2D:4D ratios in these subjects? There is some support for this in a small sample (43 males) of Jamaican boys from the Jamaican Symmetry Project. In this group 2D:4D ratio of the left hand was positively and significantly related to the birth weight recalled by the mother. There was also a positive association between 2D:4D of the right hand and birth weight, but this was not significant (left hand $b = 10.38$, $F = 4.67$, $p = 0.02$ one-tailed adjusted for multiple tests $p = 0.04$; right hand $b = 1.2$, $F = 0.04$, $p = 0.83$). One possible confound of this relationship is birth order. In a larger sample (70 males) of Jamaican boys it was found that later born boys were heavier at birth than earlier born boys (left hand $b = 0.32$, $F = 12.96$, $p = 0.0006$). A simultaneous multiple regression showed that 2D:4D of the left hand remained significantly related to birth weight after the effect of birth order was removed (2D:4D and birth weight $n = 43$, $b = 10.41$, $t = 2.11$, $p = 0.04$; birth order and birth weight $b = 0.15$, $t = 1.16$, $p = 0.25$).

It seems therefore that 2D:4D ratio may be positively associated with BW/ExBW and negatively associated with gestational age. Both findings are independent of sex. However, we must be cautious in generalizing from this conclusion because our most persuasive data relate to a special group of babies of very low birth weight. If confirmed, these results suggest that high prenatal testosterone concentrations are associated with a lower than expected birth weight and an increased gestational age in both males and females. Low birth weight children have normal IQs, but 60 to 70% experience problems at school. Many have cognitive, perceptual, and motor performance deficits. In addition many also suffer from behavioral problems sometimes called the "new morbidities." These include symptoms such as sleeping problems, lack of appetite, headache, hyperactivity, poor concentration, tendency to tire easily, and behavioral disturbances (Stevenson et al. 1999). It is possible that some of these symptoms may be associated with damage to the CNS arising from exposure to high concentrations of prenatal testosterone. More work is necessary to clarify the situation. For example, in addition to having low 2D:4D ratios, low birth weight children may also have parents with low 2D:4D. This would be further evidence that prenatal levels of androgens are important factors in the etiology of reduced growth rates in utero.

Birth Weight and Coronary Heart Disease

The fetal origins of disease is an area of research that is producing new insights into coronary heart disease. Low birth weight babies have an increased risk of death from coronary heart disease in later life (Barker 1992). One negative correlate of low birth weight is blood pressure. Elevated blood pressure is one risk factor for death from coronary heart disease. The "Seven Countries Study" is a comparative look at hypertension and its consequences in 12,761 men aged 40 to 59 years from the United States, Finland, the Netherlands, Italy, Greece, the former Yugoslavia, and Japan (Van den Hoogen et al. 2000). The study found significant differences in mean systolic and diastolic pressures between countries, and the absolute risk of death among hypertensive subjects per country varied by a factor of three to four (from 44 deaths per 10,000 person-years in Japan and the southern Mediterranean to 153 deaths per 10,000 person-years in northern Europe). However, over a 25-year period of follow-up, the relative risk of death within each country from coronary heart disease was seen to rise continuously with increasing systolic and diastolic blood pressure.

If correlates of low birth weight are positively related to 2D:4D ratio, it would appear that low 2D:4D individuals may have an increased risk of hypertension and coronary heart disease. However, there was no evidence of a negative association between 2D:4D and blood pressure in the data of Manning, Sanderson, Bundred, and Pharoah. In fact 2D:4D was positively, but not significantly, related to diastolic pressure (right hand, $b = 19.68$, $F = 1.40$, $p = 0.24$; left hand, $b = 29.92$, $F = 3.03$, $p = 0.08$).

Furthermore, although men have higher levels of mortality from coronary heart disease than women, there is evidence that testosterone is protective against myocardial infarction (heart attack) in men. This leads us to the relationship between 2D:4D ratio and the age of presentation of myocardial infarction (MI).

Myocardial Infarction

Myocardial infarction is strongly sex-dependent in its expression. Women in westernized countries have a substantially lower incidence of coronary heart disease than men. All studies of acute myocardial infarction have found that women have infarctions at older ages than men (Wexler 1999), and men are more likely to die from MI than women (e.g., for British mortality rates, see BHF 1996). When there are trends in reductions in mortality from MI this sex difference is maintained (e.g., for hospitalization and mortality from MI in the period 1987 to 1994 in the United States, see Rosamond et al. 1998). The World Health Organization's MONICA project has monitored changes in the incidence of cardiac disease in 37 populations of 21 countries for 10 years. During this period mortality from coronary heart disease declined in some countries as a result of fewer heart attacks and by the fact that heart attacks were less deadly. However, deaths in men caused by MI continued to outnumber women by four to one (Kmietowicz 1999). Important determinants of this sex difference can be found in levels of lipids and lipoproteins and in particular differences in the concentrations of high-density lipoprotein (HDL) cholesterol (Wexler 1999). In contrast, in populations with low rates of coronary heart disease there are reduced sex differences in concentrations of HDL and in mortality from MI. Geographical differences in MI incidence may correlate with 2D:4D ratios and be associated with the degree to which fetal development is "androgenized or estrogenized."

Testosterone and Heart Disease

It is a commonly held belief that testosterone tends to promote heart disease. Rosano (2000) has pointed out that this seems intuitively true because men have higher rates of coronary heart disease than women, an androgenic or malelike body fat distribution (i.e., high waist:hip ratio) is correlated with coronary artery disease in men and women, and self-administration of synthetic androgens by athletes and bodybuilders is associated with adverse changes in the lipid profile of both men and women. However, there is much evidence that endogenous testosterone is in fact a protective against heart disease in men. Animal studies have shown that testosterone replacement in castrated rabbits reduces total cholesterol and prevents atherosclerosis (Alexandersen et al. 1999), while testosterone given to female monkeys accelerates progression of atherosclerosis (Adams et al. 1995). These findings suggest that testosterone is protective against atherosclerosis in males but promotes atherosclerosis in females. In humans cross-sectional studies have found that endogenous concentrations of testosterone are positively correlated with HDL, i.e., the favorable form of cholesterol (Hamalainen et al. 1986; Barrett-Connor and Kaw 1988; Barrett-Connor 1995; Zmuda et al. 1997). Other studies have found that testosterone usually decreases with age and that this age-dependent decrease in men is associated with increases in triglycerides and a reduction in HDL cholesterol (Barrett-Connor et al. 1986; Haffner et al. 1993). A number of studies have shown that men who have had an MI tend to have low testosterone compared to healthy controls (Mendoza et al. 1983; Sewdarsen et al. 1986; Aksut et al. 1986; Swartz and Young 1987; Sewdarsen et al. 1990; Rice et al. 1993). In addition men who have had a recent MI often have higher concentrations of estrogen than controls (Entrican et al. 1978; Luria et al. 1982; Sewdarsen et al. 1986; Aksut et al. 1986; Sewdarsen et al. 1990; Cengiz et al. 1991). The important question is whether the low levels of androgens and high concentrations of estrogens in male patients with cardiovascular disease are a consequence or a cause of the disease. Experimental studies have shown testosterone to be a vasodilator when introduced into rabbit coronary arteries and aortae (Yue et al. 1995) and to be effective in promoting coronary blood flow in men (Webbet et al. 1999). In support of this English et al. (2000) have found that men with coronary artery disease have lower levels of free testosterone than controls do.

The situation in women is less clear, but there is evidence that unlike men, high testosterone and low estrogen predispose women to MI. Free testosterone has been reported to be positively associated with triglyceride concentrations, negatively with high density lipoprotein cholesterol, and positively with hypertension and coronary artery disease in women (Phillips et al. 1997). It therefore appears that testosterone and estrogen have opposite effects on the etiology of MI in men and women. It may be that these sex-dependent correlates of steroid hormones arise at the prenatal stage.

Testosterone and Prenatal Influences on Heart Disease

In the 1950s and 1960s it became apparent that populations with high mortality from cardiovascular disease tended to have high cholesterol and high blood pressure, and that obesity and smoking were common. This realization led to the "Lifestyle Model," which identified the key health issues of a low-fat diet, exercise, and abstinence from smoking. Intervention programs designed to reduce cholesterol, increase exercise, and discourage smoking did reduce rates of cardiovascular disease. However, by the mid-1980s it was apparent that lifestyle factors had a limited ability to predict cardiovascular disease in adults. For example, data from the MONICA project indicated that only 25% of the variance in cardiovascular disease was predicted by risk factors such as diet, cholesterol, smoking, and exercise (Jarvelin 2000). In the 1980s the work of Barker (1992) and his colleagues led to the realization that prenatal conditions are powerful antecedents of cardiovascular disease. This led to the concept of biological programming in fetal and infant life. The model concerns programming in utero, which may involve the effect of poor nutrition, hormones, antigens and antibodies, drugs, etc. In the case of cardiovascular disease emphasis has been placed on poor nutrition during early and mid-gestation, which, it is hypothesized, leads to an increased risk of adult disease by affecting blood pressure, cholesterol metabolism, and blood coagulation (Barker and Osmond 1986; Barker 1995). One important component in these complex associations may be the effect of sex steroids on the formation of the vascular system. First-trimester exposure to exogenous estrogen and progesterone may lead to cardiovascular anomalies, which include ventricular septal defect, atrial septal defect, pulmonic stenosis, patent ductus arteriosis, and transposition of the great vessels (Levy et al. 1973; Nora et al. 1976). It is probably not coincidental that estrogen and or progesterone treatment in the first trimester is also associated with malformations in traits under the control of Homeobox or *Hox* genes, including anomalies of the genitalia in boys and digit malformations, e.g., polydactyly, digit reduction, and fingerization of thumbs (Heinonen et al. 1977; Lorber et al. 1979).

2D:4D and Age at Myocardial Infarction

Manning and Bundred (manuscript) have investigated the association between the 2D:4D ratio and the age at presentation of first MI in men and women. Patients were recruited from the Wirral Cardiac Rehabilitation Unit of St. Catherine's Hospital, Birkenhead, in the United Kingdom. The sample consisted of 301 participants, of whom 211 were men and 90 women. There were 151 men who had experienced an MI and 54 women. Patients with angina pectoris, but with no history of MI, numbered 96 (60 men and 36 women). The preponderance of men in the sample was likely to be determined, at least in part, by the sex-dependent expression of coronary heart disease.

Male MI controls were recruited from social clubs and adult education classes in the Merseyside area. It is unlikely that 2D:4D ratio changes with age. However, the distribution of the ratio may change as a result of differential mortality. The index cases were therefore matched with controls for age in addition to sex. The age at first MI or age at first reported symptoms of angina was obtained from the patient. Height and weight were measured, and patients were asked whether they had smoked in the 12 months preceding their MI. Testosterone levels may be modulated in relation to status in mammals (Barnard et al. 1998), the incidence and prognosis of MI is related to socioeconomic status (SES) in humans (Marmot et al. 1991), and 2D:4D may be associated with SES (see chapter 2). In this instance SES was estimated by calculating the Super Profile Lifestyles classification from the patient's postal code (Brown and Batey 1987). This classification divides the population into deciles, where 1 is equal to the most affluent members of society and 10 represents the most impoverished.

There was strong evidence that men with low 2D:4D ratios had MIs at a later age than men with high ratios. The 2D:4D ratio of right and left hands and the mean 2D:4D ratio was negatively related to age at first MI (see figure 6.2). The ratio of the right hand and the mean of both hands showed significant negative relationships with age at first MI. The left-hand 2D:4D ratio was negatively but not significantly associated with age at first MI. All p values of less than 0.05 remained significant after Bonferroni adjustment for multiple tests. There was some evidence that men with lower right-hand 2D:4D than left-hand ratio (i.e., low D_{r-l}) had MIs later in life than those with high D_{r-l}, but the relationship was not significant (age at MI regressed on D_{r-l}, $b = -39.41$, $F = 2.41$, $p = 0.12$). There were weak and nonsignificant positive relationships between 2D:4D ratio and age in the controls (e.g., mean 2D:4D, $b = 43.31$, $F = 2.41$, $p = 0.12$).

As expected there was evidence that men with low Body Mass Index (BMI, kg/m^2) and high status had MIs later in life than men who were overweight and of low SES. The relationship with BMI was significant ($b = -0.82$, $F = 13.37$, $p = 0.0004$) but that of SES was not ($b = -0.47$, $F = 2.68$, $p = 0.10$). Patients who smoked in the 12 months prior to their MI ($n = 64$) had a mean age at MI of 55.68 ± 9.44 years. Nonsmokers ($n = 87$) had a significantly higher mean age (62.63 ± 10.27 years) at MI than smokers (t-test, $t = 4.08$, $p = 0.0001$). These results were consistent with known lifestyle risk factors, i.e., high BMI, low SES, and smoking, for premature MI.

The results of simultaneous multiple regression analyses with age at first MI as the dependent variable and 2D:4D ratio (right and left hand and mean), BMI, SES, and smoking habits (dummy variable; smoker = 0, nonsmoker = 1) as independent variables showed significant relationships with digit ratio (see table 6.1). The 2D:4D ratio of the right hand ($p = 0.0008$) and mean 2D:4D ($p = 0.01$) remained significant predictors of age at first MI after the effects of BMI, SES, and smoking habits were removed. It seems therefore that high 2D:4D ratio is associated with early MI in men, and the association is independent of three of the most powerful lifestyle predictors of MI, i.e., BMI, SES, and smoking.

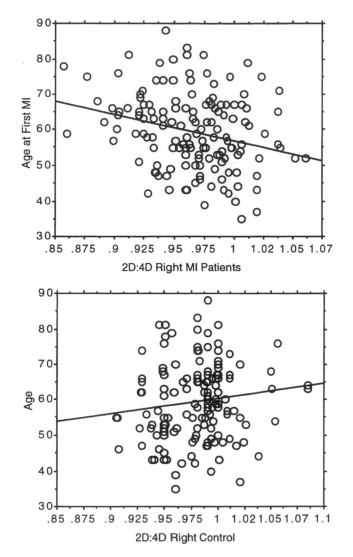

Figure 6.2. The relationship between 2D:4D ratio of the right hand and age at first MI in men. Subjects with low 2D:4D ratio have a tendency to present with their first MI later in life than men with high 2D:4D ratio (right hand $b = -75.62$, $F = 10.85$, $p = 0.001$, Bonferroni corrected $p = 0.003$; left hand $b = -35.64$, $F = 2.06$, $p = 0.15$; mean 2D:4D $b = -67.23$, $F = 5.75$, $p = 0.01$, corrected for multiple tests $p = 0.02$). In the controls (i.e., men who had not experienced an MI) there was no significant relationship with 2D:4D and age. This makes it unlikely that the 2D:4D and age at first MI association arises as the result of age related associations with 2D:4D ratio.

Table 6.1. 2D:4D ratio, BMI, SES, and smoking habits as predictors of age at first MI

Trait	beta	st. error	t	p
2D:4D right	−76.95	22.45	3.43	0.0008
BMI	−0.67	0.21	3.16	0.002
SES	−0.58	0.27	2.08	0.04
Smoking habits	6.69	1.98	3.91	0.0002
overall r^2 = 0.27				
2D:4D left	−38.93	26.80	1.45	0.15
BMI	−0.68	0.23	2.93	0.004
SES	−0.58	0.30	1.94	0.05
Smoking habits	5.88	1.98	3.25	0.002
overall r^2 = 0.19				
2D:4D mean	−72.73	29.22	2.49	0.01
BMI	−0.69	0.22	3.08	0.003
SES	−0.64	0.29	2.19	0.03
Smoking habits	6.30	1.98	3.56	0.0006
overall r^2 = 0.23				

It should be pointed out that these relationships between 2D:4D and MI are with first MIs, and, of course, with first MIs that had been survived by the patient. We do not know whether the associations are stronger or weaker when first MIs result in death. This is obviously an important question to address. It is also important to emphasize that BMI and smoking were predictors of early MIs independent of 2D:4D ratios. This means that men with low 2D:4D ratios should not assume that they are protected against the negative effects that obesity and smoking have on the heart. It is of interest in this context to note that Finns may have low 2D:4D digit ratios (see chapter 1) but they have brought down their substantial incidence of early heart attack in men by reducing consumption of saturated fats (WHO MONICA Project 1988; Kmietowicz 1999). More data is required to confirm the relationship between 2D:4D and age at first MI, but it may be particularly appropriate for men with high 2D:4D ratio to exercise regularly, to observe dietary caution, and to avoid smoking.

There was no evidence that 2D:4D ratio was correlated with age at first angina pectoris symptoms. For example, in a regression with mean 2D:4D and age at first symptoms, the slope of the line was $b = 0.80$, $F = 0.001$, $p = 0.98$. This may be because angina symptoms appear slowly over a period of time, and relationships with their age at first presentation are not readily seen. Alternatively, it may indicate that the etiology of angina and MI are not closely linked.

The female sample was smaller than that of the male, and this may have obscured real relationships. However, in common with men there was a negative (but nonsignificant) association between 2D:4D and age at first MI in women ($b = -45.55$, $F = 2.13$, $p = 0.15$). It is important to clarify whether this association is indeed real. As with men there was little evidence that 2D:4D was related to age at first angina symptoms ($b = 11.85$, $F = 0.06$, $p = 0.81$).

It is probable that, in men at least, 2D:4D ratio does tell us something about predisposition to MI. The link may begin in utero and could include associations with the formation of the vascular system that predispose to atherosclerosis and a reduction in blood flow rates. There may also be a link at the biochemical level as cholesterol is a precursor to testosterone and also an important correlate of MI. There are associations between 2D:4D ratio and waist:hip ratio. For example, a negative correlation has been reported between the waist:hip ratio of women and the 2D:4D ratio of their children (Manning et al. 1999). In addition, 2D:4D ratio is positively associated with waist:hip ratio in women (Manning, Barley et al. 2000). Waist:hip ratio is a correlate of the distribution of sites of deposition of fat around the body. In a similar way 2D:4D may be correlated with aspects of lipid metabolism and serum cholesterol levels. This link may explain associations between 2D:4D ratio and cardiovascular disease. More work is needed to clarify these and other relationships between 2D:4D and predisposition to MI.

Breast Cancer

There are a number of known risk factors for breast cancer, e.g., age, breast parenchyma type, parity, age at menarche, age at menopause. In order to understand the etiology of breast cancer one also needs to consider prenatal and adult estrogen.

Estrogen and Breast Cancer

Breast cancer is the most common cancer among women in much of the developed world (Wynder et al. 1960). Many of the postnatal risk factors are associated with increased estrogen exposure. For example, early menarche, late menopause, late first childbirth, and low parity all lead to an increase in number of lifetime ovulations. As ovulation is immediately preceded by a surge in estrogen, these factors increase lifetime exposure to estrogen and predispose to presentation of breast cancer (Kelsey and

Berkowitz 1986; Brinton et al. 1988). Breast asymmetry may also increase with mid-cycle changes in breast size caused by estrogen production (Manning et al. 1997), and breast asymmetry may be positively correlated with breast cancer (Scutt et al. 1997). Treatment of breast cancer is based on the association between estrogen and growth and proliferation of the tumor. Estrogen receptors are found in 50 to 80% of breast tumors. Endocrine treatments antagonize the effects of estrogen. Reduction of estrogen concentrations may be obtained by oophorectemy, luteinizing hormone-releasing hormone agonists, and aromatase inhibition. Alternatively the binding of estrogen to cell receptors may be blocked by anti-estrogens such as tamoxifen. Of those metastatic tumors that test positive to estrogen receptors, some 50 to 60% respond to endocrine treatments, while of those that are negative for receptors less than 5% respond (Elledge and Osborne 1997).

Estrogen may precipitate breast cancer because it stimulates proliferation of the breast epithelium, thus predisposing to cancer initiation (Anderson et al. 1989). Geographical differences in breast cancer rates may be partly explainable in terms of differences in estrogen concentrations. For example, Asian women have lower levels of breast cancer and serum estrogen than have Western women (Key et al. 1990). Migration to the West is also associated with increases in breast cancer rates and estrogen concentration in women of Chinese and Japanese origin (Trichopoulos et al. 1984). Postnatal factors are unable to explain the striking international differences in incidence rates of breast cancer. For example, Caucasian women in the United States and the United Kingdom have five times higher incidence than Oriental women in China and Japan (Kelsey and Berkowitz 1986; Trichopoulos 1990).

Trichopoulos (1990) has argued that exposure to prenatal estrogen may explain much of the within- and between-population variance of breast cancer incidence. He pointed out that (a) estrogens are important in breast carcinogenesis; (b) postnatal factors that increase the probability of cancer may also act prenatally; (c) estrogen concentrations are 10 or more times higher during pregnancy than at other times; and (d) during pregnancy estrogen secretion varies widely among individuals.

In order to test Trichopoulos's theory we need a sensitive proxy for prenatal estrogen. High birth weight has been suggested as a surrogate for high prenatal estrogen. Sanderson et al. (1996) have found that women with a birth weight of greater than 4,000 g were at increased risk of breast cancer. There is evidence that high birth weight is associated with high 2D:4D ratios. Subject recall of birth weight may be inaccurate or not available. The 2D:4D ratio could provide a more reliable indicator of breast cancer, and one that is correlated with age at presentation of the tumor.

2D:4D Ratios and Breast Cancer

The 2nd and 4th digits of the right and left hands of a sample of 118 women who had presented with breast cancer were measured in the Royal Liverpool Hospital (Manning and Leinster 2001). The mean age of the patients was 56 ± 11.47 years. Breast cancer expression is strongly age-dependent. In the initial sample a number of the participants had deformities of the digits associated with arthritis and other conditions. These subjects were excluded from the study. Controls, matched for sex and age, were recruited from social clubs and adult education classes in the Merseyside area.

There was evidence that women with low 2D:4D ratios (i.e., who may have had low prenatal and postpubertal estrogen) presented with breast cancer later in life than women with high 2D:4D ratios. Unlike the MI sample, the relationship was significant in the left hand but not the right (see figure 6.3). As with the MI sample the mean 2D:4D ratio was significantly related to age at cancer presentation ($b = -94.49$, $F = 6.71$, $p = 0.01$). Correction for multiple tests left the mean and left-hand associations significant. Controls showed weak positive relationships between 2D:4D ratio and age of subjects that were nonsignificant (mean 2D:4D, $b = 52.3$, $F = 2.36$, $p = 0.13$).

I interpret these results to support the hypothesis that women with high 2D:4D ratio (i.e., with high prenatal estrogen) may have a tendency to present early with breast cancer. Further work is needed to confirm this result. If the finding is proved to be robust, we also need to know whether 2D:4D is a stronger risk factor for breast cancer than other well-established risks. The 2D:4D ratio may make more accurate the identification of women for whom early screening is desirable. More work is needed before we can reach this stage.

Hypotheses

The use of 2D:4D ratios to identify high-risk groups may be possible for a number of diseases (Manning and Bundred 2000).

Diabetes and 2D:4D Ratio

The 2D:4D ratio may be related to the etiology of diabetes, particularly diabetes that is non-insulin dependent (NIDDM). Diabetes is a risk factor for MI and many of its effects are vascular (Haffner et al. 1999). NIDDM or type II diabetes is dependent on waist circumference, waist:hip ratio, and BMI in both men and women (Wei et al. 1997). However, in men upper body adiposity is related to low androgenicity, while in women it is correlated with high concentrations of androgens. There is some evidence

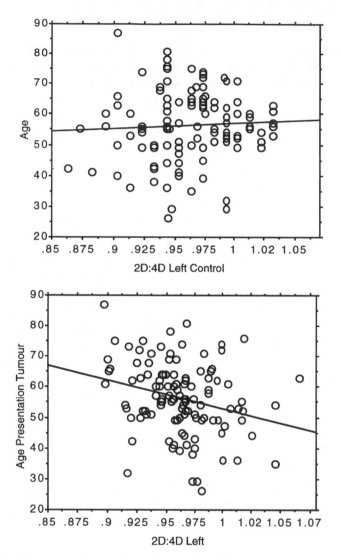

Figure 6.3. The relationship between 2D:4D ratio of the left hand and age at first presentation of a malignant breast tumor in 118 women. The association was significant for the left hand ($b = -95.27$, $F = 8.74$, $p = 0.004$, corrected for multiple tests $p = 0.008$), but not the right hand ($b = -52.80$, $F = 2.56$, $p = 0.11$). The women with high 2D:4D ratios (i.e., evidence of high prenatal exposure to estrogen) were on average younger at first presentation of the breast tumor than women with low 2D:4D ratio (i.e., evidence of low prenatal exposure to estrogen). There was no significant relationship between age and 2D:4D ratio in a control sample matched for sex and age (e.g., mean 2D:4D $b = 52.30$, $F = 2.36$, $p = 0.13$).

that high levels of free testosterone are associated with decreased insulin concentrations in men but increased insulin levels in women (for review, see Haffner 1996). These associations suggest that high 2D:4D in men and low 2D:4D in women may be predictive of NIDDM.

Prostate Cancer and 2D:4D Ratio

The 2D:4D ratio may be useful in the identification of high-risk groups in relation to cancers of the reproductive system, e.g., prostate, endometrial, and ovarian carcinomas. Testosterone and its principal metabolite dihydrotestosterone are the major trophic factors that regulate growth and function of epithelial prostate tissue. Ross et al. (1986) have pointed out that African Americans have the highest rate of prostate cancer in the world, and nearly twice that of whites in the United States. After adjustment for lifestyle factors, they found that a sample of African American students had a 15% higher total testosterone level than white students. They concluded that the magnitude of the difference in testosterone concentration is sufficient to explain a twofold difference in prostate cancer risk. Men with low 2D:4D may be susceptible to early presentation of prostate cancer. In this context it would be of interest to know whether concentrations of prostate-specific antigen (PSA), a correlate of division rate in prostate epithelia, is related to 2D:4D ratio in middle-aged and elderly men. High levels of PSA may be associated with low 2D:4D ratio after the effect of age is removed.

Ovarian and Endometrial Cancers and 2D:4D Ratio

A review of factors affecting women's reproductive cancers (Boyd et al. 1994) has shown that early menarche, low parity, and late menopause are predictive of endometrial and ovarian cancers. All these factors increase lifetime exposure to estrogen. Women in westernized countries tend to have lower parity and less breastfeeding experience than women from traditional societies. The former may therefore be disposed to estrogen-dependent cancers of the reproductive system because they have many more ovulations than the latter. In common with patients with breast cancer, women with high 2D:4D ratios may have earlier presentation of both endometrial and ovarian tumors.

The Immune System, HIV/AIDS, and 2D:4D Ratio

The 2D:4D ratio may correlate with patterns of immune disorders. Geschwind and Galaburda (1985a, 1985b, 1985c) have pointed out that the pattern of immune disorders is strongly sex-dependent. Before puberty the allergic disorders such as asthma, eczema, and hay fever are

more strongly expressed in boys. Prenatal testosterone may predispose to
such allergies. It may be fruitful to examine 2D:4D ratios in patients with
these diseases. Low 2D:4D ratios may be predictive of susceptibility. After
puberty testosterone suppresses the immune system so that autoimmune
diseases are more common in females than in males. These postpubertal
autoimmune diseases may be associated with high 2D:4D. However, this
also means that postpubertal females are more immunocompetent than
males. There is therefore a male predominance of cancers and a female
predominance of autoimmune disease. Experimental work with mice
(Kimura et al. 1995) has shown sex differences in the concentrations of T
cells in various organs. Autoimmunity is at least partly dependent on
the activation of self-recognizing T cells. The liver in female mice has
large numbers of T cells with T cell receptor cells. Male mice have fewer
numbers of self-recognizing T cells. Removal of the testes caused an increase in such cells and exogenous testosterone removes this consequence
of castration.

Susceptibility to viruses such as HIV and progression to symptoms of
AIDS may be related to high prenatal testosterone, i.e., low 2D:4D ratio.
This is an emotive topic, but it would be of great value if we could identify individuals susceptible to HIV infection and therefore make advice on
safe sex and the supply of condoms more effective. In 1998 20 million
people died of AIDS, and in 1999 it became the world's leading infectious
disease killer.

At the beginning of the AIDS pandemic HIV/AIDS was initially largely
associated with homosexual transmission between men. Now infection is
predominantly heterosexual and centered on sub-Saharan Africa, and 67%
of people with HIV/AIDS are in this area (Gilks 1999). Within southern
Africa life expectancy has been cut by a quarter, infection rates and rates
of vertical transmission are high, patients with AIDS-related infections
occupy 70% of hospital beds, and rates of tuberculosis associated with AIDS
are increasing (Logie 1999; Kleinschmidt 1999; LePage and Day 2000;
Grimwood 2000). This pattern may be related to testosterone.

Geschwind and Galaburda (1985a) have argued that gay men are
exposed to higher concentrations of prenatal testosterone than heterosexuals. Masculinization of external genitalia begins at 7 weeks of gestation, and if testosterone is not present until 12 weeks, full development
cannot occur (Migeon and Wisniewski 1998). Bogaert and Hershberger
(1999) have reported that gay men often have greater development of the
penis than heterosexuals. There are also some reports of higher testosterone concentrations in homosexual men compared to heterosexuals
(Brodie et al. 1974; Doerr et al. 1976; Friedman et al. 1977). Of course

the strongest predictor of HIV status is sexual behavior. It may be the case that low 2D:4D is correlated with high sex drive and number of lifetime sexual partners. If so any relationship between 2D:4D ratio and the etiology of sexually transmitted diseases is likely to be reinforced. Number of lifetime sexual partners may be higher in homosexual men than in heterosexuals (Gorman 1984). Robinson and Manning (2000) have found that homosexual men have lower 2D:4D ratios than heterosexuals, suggesting higher prenatal testosterone in the former compared to the latter.

In contrast to Western countries the transmission of HIV is predominantly heterosexual in southern Africa. Black South Africans have very low 2D:4D ratios, and South Africa has 10% of the world's AIDS population (LePage and Day 2000). The association between low 2D:4D, male homosexuality, and the ethnic and geographical pattern of HIV/AIDS may indicate that individuals with low 2D:4D are susceptible to both horizontal and vertical transmission of the virus. Such transmission is less probable in populations with high 2D:4D ratio such as in Poland, Spain, and England. It is likely that HIV-1 had its origins in a virus that normally infects chimpanzees. The less common HIV-2 may have come from sooty mangabeys (Bailey 2000). The species jump is likely to have occurred when infected primates were hunted for meat. However, Hooper (2000) has controversially argued that HIV could have been transmitted to humans through infected polio vaccines distributed in Central Africa in the 1950s. There are a number of problems with Hooper's thesis. For example, there were in fact two large distributions of the polio vaccine, one in Africa and the other in Poland. It may be merely coincidence but the Poles have one of the lowest rates of HIV infection in Europe and the highest mean 2D:4D ratio thus far measured. It could be profitable to look for correlations between population 2D:4D ratios and HIV infection rates. This may be best done in southern Africa where infection rates are generally high but show considerable geographical heterogeneity.

Parasitic Infections and 2D:4D Ratios

Grossman (1989) has summarized evidence that immune mechanisms show considerable sexual dimorphism in humans. Two important components of the immune response are the production of antibody molecules by B cells and cell-mediated immunity associated with the activity of T cells (Staines et al. 1992). Grossman (1989) suggested that sex steroids affect the development of the immune system during early fetal development. He summarized evidence that sex steroids act at the level of stem cells, pre-T and pre-B lymphocytes, and on fetal thymic tissue. These effects then lead on to sexual dimorphisms in immune function in adults.

The most compelling evidence for sexually dimorphic immune responses is in the circulating concentrations of antibodies. An antibody molecule is Y-shaped. The stem of the molecule is the C region, and it is variation in this region that is used to classify the major groups of antibodies (Staines et al. 1992). The major classes are IgG, which protects the extravascular space from microorganisms and their toxins; IgM, which is a first line of defense against microorganisms in the bloodstream; and IgD, which protects mucosal surfaces. Circulating concentrations of these major immunoglobulin classes are lower in males than in females of the same age (Butterworth et al. 1967; Rowe et al. 1968). These findings are consistent with reports of males mounting lower antibody responses than females to polio (Ainbender et al. 1968), *Escherichia coli* (Michaels and Rogers 1971), measles (Patty et al. 1967), rubella (Spencer et al. 1977), brucella (Rhodes et al. 1969), and hepatitis B (London and Drew 1977). The evidence for sex differences in the cell-mediated response is less convincing. However, Grossman (1989) has considered evidence that females have a more active response, and this is supported by reports of a lowered incidence of tumors and superior resistance to viral and parasitic infections in females compared to males.

Brabin and Brabin (1992) have provided an excellent review of sexual dimorphisms in parasite prevalence, density, and disease manifestation. There are marked sex differences in host response to many infections of great public health concern. These include lymphatic filariasis and onchocerciasis leading to river blindness and elephantiasis; protozoal infections leading to Chagas' disease, sleeping sickness; visceral leishmaniasis resulting in kala azar; and malaria parasites facilitating the development of Burkitt's lymphoma and splenomegaly. Onchocerciasis may be used to illustrate the serious nature of many of these diseases (WHO 1987). The causative agent of onchocerciasis is the tissue-dwelling nematode *Onchocerca volvulus*. The nematode is spread via infected *Simulium* (blackfly or buffalo fly) vectors. Adult female worms are found in nodules in the human host. Each worm may produce 3,000 microfilariae per day, and the average fertile life span is 9 to 11 years. The microfilariae cause itching, loss of skin color, rapid aging, and victims often become blind by their mid-thirties. The disease is found in sub-Saharan Africa, Yemen, and in parts of Central and South America. It is particularly prevalent in fertile land around rapidly flowing rivers. As a result many potentially productive valleys cannot be cultivated due to the severity of the disease. This is particularly problematic in the Sahel region of Africa, because these fertile areas are urgently needed to provide food to a malnourished population. Infected people have reduced productivity, and their ability to provide resources for their children is seriously impaired. Approximately one million people are substantially sight-impaired or blind because of onchocerciasis, and 40,000 new cases of blindness occur each year in Africa. There may be up to 17 million people currently infected, and over 100 million remain at risk of infection. Control of onchocerciasis and other diseases caused by parasites is therefore of great importance. Many of these infections show a pattern of higher susceptibility in males. *The important point to make here is that low values of 2D:4D in both males and females may be predictive of susceptibility to these parasites.*

Males have a greater prevalence of infection for lymphatic filariasis. Brabin (1990) reviewed 53 studies from Africa, Asia, the Indian subcontinent, and the Americas, and found 43 showed higher mean prevalence of infection in males. Clinical manifestations of disease were also more intense in males than in females. These included filarial fevers and acute lymphangitis in areas endemic for *Wuchereria bancrofti*, and elephantiasis in areas endemic for *Brugia malayi*. For *Onchocerca volvulus* microfilarial densities are often greater in males than females (Brandling-Bennett et al. 1981). The sex difference in worm loads can be seen from the age of five years in West Africa and earlier in Central America. The intensity of infection is known to be related to the severity of ocular onchocerciasis. Ocular lesions and blindness are more common in males.

There appears to be no sex difference in parasitaemia from infection with *Trypanosoma cruzi*. However, lesions associated with chronic heart disease and megaesophagus often occur more frequently in men (Oliviera et al. 1981; Mota et al. 1984). Similarly, a longitudinal study of Chagas disease in central Brazil found electrocardiogram alterations and left anterior hemiblock to be more common in males (Zicker et al. 1990). Flagellates of the genus *Leishmania* attack the endothelial cells in blood vessels. Sex differences in visceral leishmaniasis are common, and a number of studies of kala azar have found it to be more common in boys than girls. A similar pattern of male preponderance has been found for visceral leishmaniasis in East Africa and China (Brabin and Brabin 1992). An excess of male patients compared to females is seen in Burkitt's lymphoma. This is a cancer associated with malaria and infection with Epstein-Barr virus. The lymphoma is thought to be caused by malarial infection of individuals with the virus. In Papua, New Guinea, Burkitt and O'Connor (1961) found a male:female ratio of 2:1, while Reay-Young and Chir (1974) reported a similar ratio of 1.8:1. Infection with *Plasmodium* may disorder the host's immune system and lead to neoplastic expression. If so, the effect on the immune system is more marked in males. African trypanosomiasis has also been considered a disease in which males predominate (Veatch

1946; Robertson 1963). However, there remains some doubt over this conclusion (Brabin and Brabin 1992).

It may be that an excess of males for some of these diseases can be in part explained by sex-dependent behavioral differences leading to a higher exposure of males or females to the parasite. We must not neglect this possible explanation. However, it is probable that this does not entirely explain the sex-dependent pattern of expression (Brabin and Brabin 1992). In many cases 2D:4D ratio could be predictive of disease risk. Low values of 2D:4D, i.e., malelike ratios, may indicate high-risk individuals. If so, this could be used as a screening tool that would enable more effective application of public health initiatives. For example, in onchocerciasis the drug ivermectin is used to reduce the infective pool of microfilariae. It may be more effective if its use is particularly directed toward both males and females with low values of 2D:4D ratio.

A greater susceptibility of disease risk in females can sometimes be found. For example, there is a general opinion that malaria parasite prevalence is similar in males and females. However, an important exception is that females experience increased susceptibility to malaria in their first pregnancies. There are substantial implications for this observation because malaria tends to reduce fetal growth rate in primiparae compared to multiparae (Brabin 1991). The effect leads to an increase in risk for low birth weight (i.e., less than 2,500 g) in primiparae in areas endemic for malaria of between 10 to 40%. The mechanism underlying the risk of malaria for primiparae is unknown. One possibility is that the increase in estrogen concentrations during pregnancy has a suppressive effect on immune function. In support of this Kita et al. (1989) found that nonspecific immune responses were suppressed by estrogen. It could be that high estrogen production in pregnancy is associated with high values of 2D:4D. Therefore, in areas endemic for malaria primiparae with high 2D:4D may be particularly susceptible to malaria.

Conclusions

The data presented in this chapter indicate that high values of 2D:4D ratio may be correlated with early MI in men and early presentation of breast cancer in women. Low 2D:4D may be associated with a slowing of in utero development in both sexes. Diseases such as type II diabetes; prostate, endometrial, and ovarian cancers; HIV/AIDS; and various important parasitic infections may also be related to patterns of 2D:4D ratio.

There are many other instances of sex-dependent differences in disease expression (e.g., cancer of the lung and colon are more common in men), and in the reaction to many drugs (see Geschwind and Galaburda 1985a, 1985c, 1985c, and Brabin and Brabin 1992 for reviews). Prenatal testosterone could correlate with the expression of such traits. Of course, the incidence of some of these diseases is associated with cigarette smoking, alcohol consumption, and dietary habits. We do not yet know whether high prenatal testosterone predisposes individuals to "risk-taking behaviors" such as smoking, alcoholism, drug addiction, dietary excess, etc. Studies of 2D:4D ratios and these behaviors may yield important evidence for the etiology of disease.

CHAPTER 7

Male and Female Homosexuality

What is the mechanism that establishes sexual orientation in humans? How does selection operate on this mechanism? These are important questions, because heterosexual orientation is itself a very relevant component of direct fitness. Put another way, homosexuality reduces lifetime reproductive success. For example, in one study adult male homosexuals reported about one-fifth the number of children as male heterosexuals (Bell, Weinberg, and Hammersmith 1981). Therefore, an erotic attraction to same-sex partners is difficult to explain by invoking adaptationist interpretations of behavior. The problem is compounded by the lack of evidence for nonbiological explanations for homosexual behavior. A cross-cultural survey by Stoller and Herdt (1985) provided little evidence that sexual orientation is the product of conditioning in adolescence. Similarly, the psychodynamic hypothesis that male homosexuals tend to be distant from their fathers shows small effect sizes (Bell et al. 1981). Clearly the notions that homosexuality is an illness or a sign of moral weakness or that gay men learn to be that way are not supported by empirical work.

Homosexuality, Genes, and Neurohormonal Influences

In contrast there is now a great deal of evidence to support a role for genetic and neurohormonal influences on the etiology of male homosexuality. Brothers of homosexual men are about four times more likely to be homosexual than brothers of heterosexuals (Pillard and Weinrich 1987). Studies of twins have found a dizygotic concordance rate of 15% (Kallman 1952) and 22% (Bailey and Pillard 1991) in comparison to monozygotic concordance scores of 40% (Heston and Shields 1968) and 52% (Bailey and Pillard 1991). As expected, heritability estimates are high under a variety of genetic models ($h^2 = 0.31$ to $h^2 = 0.74$; Bailey and Pillard 1991). Hamer et al. (1993) and Hu et al. (1995) have provided further support for a genetic influence on the gay phenotype when their analyses of the long arm of the X chromosome (Xq28) indicated linkage between Xq28 markers and male homosexuality.

The neurohormonal theory of sexual orientation is one mechanism that may provide a link between genes and the homosexual male phenotype. Prenatal exposure to testosterone can masculinize sexual behavior in rodents and primates (Hodgkin 1991; Pilgrim and Reisert 1992). This evidence from animal models has influenced constitutional theories of human sexuality. Such theories have emphasized the organizing role of testosterone in the prenatal masculinization and defeminization of the brain. Support for this model comes from reports that homosexual males often have female-orientated cognitive abilities in those tasks that show gender-dependent scores (Sanders and Ross-Field 1986) and from work on neuroendocrine activity in males with different sexual orientations (Dorner et al. 1975).

Before discussing empirical evidence for how sexual orientation is determined, a few definitions may clarify issues (see Migeon and Wisniewski 1998 for a review of sexual differentiation, including definitions relating to gender and sexual orientation). The gender of an individual is the sex that that person identifies with. Gender role is the sex others assign to an individual. We are concerned here with sexual orientation. Erotic attraction or sexual orientation toward members of the same sex is homosexuality, toward the opposite sex it is heterosexuality, and toward both sexes it is bisexuality. Bisexuality appears to be rare, and the distribution of heterosexual and homosexual preferences is probably polymorphic, i.e., two distinct groups with few overlaps. The frequency of homosexuality is quite high. It is unlikely to be maintained by mutation pressure alone. The prevalence of male homosexuality in Westernized societies is 1 to 4%, and there is little evidence that it is different in other groups (Bell et al. 1981; LeVay 1993; Hamer and Copeland 1994).

Gender identity and gender role are usually concordant with sex of rearing. However, there are both men and women who are discordant for both gender identity and gender role. For example, a man who is discordant for gender identity views himself as a female, and a man who assumes the role of a woman is discordant for gender role.

Congenital adrenal hyperplasia (CAH) provides an opportunity to investigate issues of gender in females who are concordant for genetic sex and mullerian duct development, but who have had high prenatal exposure to androgens and have ambiguous or masculinized genitalia (see Migeon and Wisniewski 1998 for review). Females with CAH have low levels of cortisol and high concentrations of adrenal androgens. This leads to the masculinization of external genitalia.

There is little evidence that CAH females have a conflict with their female identity. However, they may show masculinized play behavior and in some studies increased bisexual and homosexual fantasy and behavior. Variability is a characteristic of the expression of these behaviors in CAH females. Migeon and Wisniewski (1998) have speculated that this may have its origin in variation in concentrations of prenatal androgens, or in the masculinization of the genitalia or effectiveness of reconstructive surgery.

In males complete androgen insensitivity leads to female external genitalia and breast development. A feminine gender role and gender identity is typical of such males, despite levels of testosterone that are within the normal male range (Money et al. 1984).

Prenatal androgen concentrations may influence sexual orientation through early brain organization. Geschwind and Galaburda (1985a, 1985b) have pointed out that male gays have higher frequencies of left-handedness and more immune disorders than heterosexuals. This may mean that male homosexuals have been exposed to higher prenatal concentrations of androgens than heterosexual males. Alternatively, the timing of the prenatal peak of testosterone may be different in male homosexuals and heterosexuals. There are some reports of higher concentrations of testosterone in male gays compared to heterosexual men (Brodie et al. 1974; Doerr et al. 1976; Friedman et al. 1977). There is evidence that various measures of penis length and circumference (total sample of about 4,200 men) indicate that penis size may be greater in gay men compared to heterosexuals (Bogaert and Hershberger 1999). Evidence for hypermasculinization of both homosexual men and women extends also to sex differences in the human auditory system. Females have greater hearing sensitivity, greater susceptibility to noise exposure at high frequencies, more spontaneous otoacoustic emissions (OAEs), and stronger click-evoked emissions (McFadden 1998). OAEs are sounds generated by normal cochleas and emitted back through the middle ear into the external ear canal where they can be detected using small microphone systems (McFadden and Pasanen 1999). The sex-dependent pattern of more spontaneous OAEs and stronger click-evoked OAEs in women than men is found in infants and children (Burns et al. 1992; Norton 1992) and remains reasonably constant throughout life (Burns et al. 1994). It has been reported that females with male co-twins have similar OAEs to males with or without twins. This has reasonably been interpreted as the result of androgen derived from the male twin and its masculinization effect on the auditory system of the female co-twin (McFadden 1993). The pattern of click-evoked and spontaneous OAEs in both male and female homosexuals is consistent with a greater masculinization of the auditory system in gays compared to heterosexuals (McFadden and Pasanen 1999; McFadden and Champlin 2000). Evidence of this kind suggests that in individuals with low prenatal androgen there is a sexual preference for men, an increase in androgen results in a preference for women, and a further increase predisposes to a preference for men (McFadden and Champlin 2000).

In contrast to the evidence that homosexuals are hypermasculinized, there is an indication that male gays may have a partially female-differentiated brain. In heterosexual men injections of estradiol lead to a low response in the production of luteinizing hormone, while in hetero-sexual women the response is strong. Homosexual men have been re-ported to show an intermediate level response in luteinizing hormone (Dorner et al. 1975; Gladue et al. 1984). These data have been challenged (Gooren 1986; Hendricks et al. 1989), and the estradiol-luteinizing hormone relationship in homosexual men remains unresolved. Never-theless, drawing on the evidence from animal studies, MacCulloch and Waddington (1981) have suggested that low levels of prenatal androgens are the critical factor in the determination of male homosexuality. More evidence of the involvement of low concentrations of prenatal testoster-one in the gay male phenotype comes from studies of gender-dependent cognitive abilities. Tests of visuo-spatial performance, e.g., versions of the water-level task and hemifield dot detection, have shown that homosexual males have scores that resemble those from heterosexual females rather than heterosexual males (Sanders and Ross-Field 1986). In addition, in-dications that a prenatal influence of androgen is important for sexual orientation in men comes from the work of Hall and Kimura (1994). They found that dermatoglyphic asymmetry was sex-dependent in its pattern and that male gays had an intermediate pattern to heterosexual males and females.

2D:4D and Male Homosexuality

Because there is indirect evidence that implicates both high and low con-centrations of androgens in male homosexuality, a consideration of 2D:4D ratios in heterosexuals and homosexuals may help to distinguish between these alternatives.

An English Sample

Robinson and Manning (2000) have tested these ideas in a sample of male gays. The length of the 2nd and 4th digits was measured on the left and right hands of 91 English men who described themselves as homosexual, gay, or bisexual. Three of the subjects had injuries to one hand, reducing our sample to 88 participants. Mean age was 30.43 ± 9.22 years with a range of 18 to 67 years. The subjects were asked to indicate on a seven-point scale (0 = never to 6 = always) their response which most closely represented their own behavior with regard to the following statements: (a) your past sexual partners have been men; (b) this year's sexual episodes have been with men; (c) when fantasizing alone you think of men; (d) when fantasizing during sex you think of men; (e) the people you say that you fancy are men; (f) those that you try/tried to chat up are men. The distri-bution of the mean sexual orientation score per subject was skewed toward exclusive homosexuality (mean score = 5.65 ± 0.57, range 3 to 6). Half of the subjects reported scores of six (n = 44); that is, they were exclusively homosexual in their partners and their fantasies. The remainder reported sexual experiences and/or fantasies involving women.

The mean 2D:4D of the homosexual sample was 0.97 ± 0.03 for the right and 0.96 ± 0.03 for the left hand. The sample was matched for sex and age from men in the general Liverpool population; i.e., recruitment was without regard to sexual orientation. The controls had a mean 2D:4D ratio of 0.98 ± 0.04 for both right and left hands. This was very similar to reported means for Liverpool men (e.g., Manning et al. 1998). Homosexual men had a significantly lower 2D:4D ratio than population norms for the left hand (see figure 7.1). There was also a lower 2D:4D ratio in the right hand of homosexuals but the difference was not significant (t = 1.38, p = 0.17). An increase in size of the male homosexual sample to 141 participants gave similar 2D:4D ratios (0.97 ± 0.03 for right and left hands; Manning and Robinson, manuscript). These mean ratios were significantly lower than mean 2D:4D (0.98 ± 0.04) from a normative male sample of 742 Caucasians from the Liverpool area of the United Kingdom (right hand t = 2.48, p = 0.01; left hand t = 3.70, p = 0.0002). The observation that 2D:4D is lower in homosexual men than population norms is in accord with the ideas of Geschwind and Galaburda (1985a, 1985b) that homosexual men have experienced high prenatal testosterone.

However, within the homosexual sample subjects that had high sexual orientation scores (i.e., they tended to be exclusively homosexual) had high 2D:4D ratios. Thus there was a positive and significant relationship between 2D:4D and base-10 log Sexual Orientation Score in the right and left hand. Removing the exclusively homosexual men (n = 44) made little difference to the strength and direction of the relationship (see figure 7.2).

Much of the relationship between 2D:4D and sexual orientation resided in the length of the 4th digit. There was a negative association between the mean length of the ring finger of the right and left hands divided by height and base-10 log sexual orientation score (b = –0.63, F = 6.32, p = 0.01, Bonferonni adjustment p = 0.02). That is, homosexual men with short ring fingers tended to be exclusively homosexual. There was no relationship between the base-10 log sexual orientation score and 2nd digit length divided by height (b = 0.26, F = 0.83, p = 0.36). However, digit length corrected for height was positively related to age for both the 2nd and the 4th digit (mean 2D b = 152.27, F = 9.87, p = 0.002; mean 4D b = 124.62, F = 7.58, p = 0.007). Most gay men have accepted their sexual orientation by age 18, but some have not (Bell et al. 1981, 99). Therefore, younger gay men may be less sure of their sexuality than older homosexual men. Age was not significantly related to the log transformed sexual orientation score ($b = 0.001$, $F = 2.69$, $p = 0.10$). A simultaneous multiple regression analysis with mean 2D/height, mean 4D/height, and age as independent variables and log transformed sexual orientation score as the dependent variable showed that mean 4D/height remained as a significant negative predictor of sexual orientation ($b = -1.35$, $t = 3.29$, $p = 0.002$). Age was positively related to sexual orientation; i.e., older homosexuals

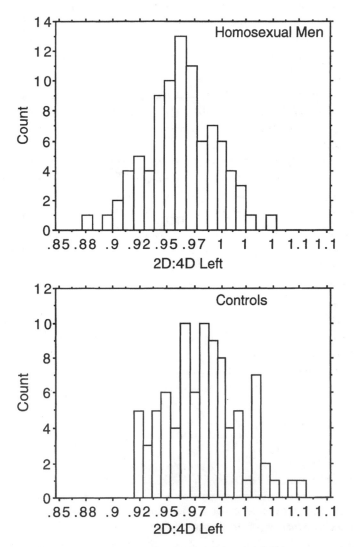

Figure 7.1. The distribution of 2D:4D ratio in the left hands of 88 homosexual men and 88 men recruited without regard to sexual orientation. Note that the homosexual sample has 2D:4D ratios shifted toward low values compared to controls (unpaired t test, $t = 3.82$, $p = 0.0002$, Bonferroni adjustment for multiple tests $p = 0.004$).

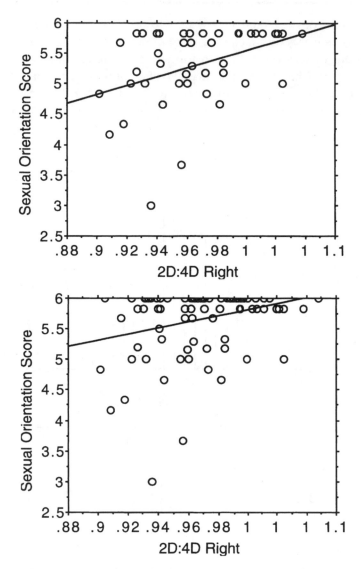

Figure 7.2. The relationship between 2D:4D ratio of the right hand and sexual orientation score (right hand $b = 0.43$, $F = 7.14$, $p = 0.009$, Bonferroni adjustment $p = 0.02$; left hand $b = 0.37$, $F = 5.05$, $p = 0.03$) in a sample of 88 men with scores from 3 to 6 (where 3 = bisexuality and 6 = an exclusively homosexual phenotype) and the sample when the exclusively gay men have been removed ($n = 44$, right hand $b = 0.64$, $F = 7.25$, $p = 0.01$, Bonferroni correction $p = 0.02$; left hand $b = 0.64$, $F = 5.69$, $p = 0.02$). Both samples show an increase in homosexuality with an increase in 2D:4D ratio.

were more likely to be exclusively gay ($b = 0.001$, $t = 2.11$, $p = 0.04$) while 2D/height was not associated with sexual orientation ($b = 0.64$, $t = 1.45$, $p = 0.15$). The data indicate that within this group who regard themselves as gay, homosexual, or bisexual, the men with high 2D:4D ratio and short 4th digit length corrected for height tend to behave in an exclusively homosexual way.

Consider now the complete sample, i.e., controls, the exclusively homosexual men, and the nonexclusively homosexual men (total $n = 176$). The controls had the highest 2D:4D ratio (right and left hand 0.98 ± 0.04), with lower 2D:4D in exclusively homosexual men (right and left hand 0.97 ± 0.03) and the lowest ratios in the nonexclusively homosexual sample (right hand 0.97 ± 0.04 and left hand 0.96 ± 0.03). The differences were significant in the left hand but not in the right (ANOVA, $F = 1.05$, $p = 0.35$). These data support an association between male homosexuality and high fetal testosterone (see figure 7.3). Very high testosterone concentrations may be associated with a sexual preference for men and women.

Before we leave this study it is of interest to consider the pattern of handedness in the sample. It is often said that gay men have an increased incidence of left-handedness compared to heterosexuals (Geschwind and Galaburda 1985a, 1985b). Could left-handedness be a predictor of sexual orientation? Manning, Trivers et al. (2000) reported low 2D:4D and low

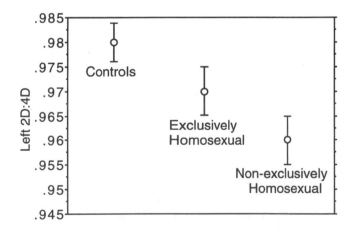

Figure 7.3. The mean 2D:4D ratios of the left hand and their standard errors for a control group of 88 men recruited without regard to their sexual orientation, a sample of 44 men who were exclusively homosexual, and 44 nonexclusively homosexual men. The controls had higher 2D:4D ratio than the homosexual men, and the lowest ratios were found in the nonexclusively homosexual men (ANOVA, $F = 7.43$, $p = 0.0008$, Bonferonni adjusted $p = 0.002$; right hand $F = 1.05$, $p = 0.35$).

D_{r-l} were related to a left-hand preference in a peg-moving task. That is, individuals with relatively long 4th digits compared to their 2nd and lower 2D:4D ratio in the right hand compared to the left were more likely to show a left-hand preference. In the sample of 91 gay men there were 16 (18%) who reported themselves as left-handed and 75 (82%) who claimed to be right-handed. There was a nonsignificant tendency for the left-handers to have lower 2D:4D (mean 0.96 ± 0.03) than the right-handers (mean 0.97 ± 0.03, Mann-Whitney U test Z-corrected for ties $= 1.45$, $p = 0.15$) and a significant tendency for a lower D_{r-l} in left-handers (mean -0.012) than right-handers (mean 0.008, Mann-Whitney U test Z-corrected for ties $= 2.27$, $p = 0.02$). A quantitative estimate of hand preference was assessed using a modified version of the Edinburgh Scale of Hand Preference. Participants reported their preferred hand in writing, throwing, holding a toothbrush, the upper hand on a broom, opening a box, drawing, using scissors, using a knife without a fork, striking a match, using a spoon, and their foot preference for kicking and eye preference when using only one. The proportion of right–sided activities per participant was assessed from this questionnaire. As predicted, there was a positive relationship between base-10 log transformed proportion of right-handedness and both mean 2D:4D and D_{r-l}. The relationships were weak, but as the direction of the associations had been predicted we used one-tailed tests. The association between handedness and D_{r-l} was significant (mean 2D:4D $b = 13.61$, $F = 2.41$, $p = 0.06$ one-tailed; $D_{r-l} b = 8.92$, $F = 3.6$, $p = 0.03$ one-tailed). The sexual orientation score was not significantly associated with proportion of right-handedness, nor was it higher for left-handers compared with right-handers. A multiple regression analysis showed the relationship between mean 2D:4D and base-10 log transformed sexual orientation score remained significant after the effect of handedness (dummy coded left $= 1$ and right $= 2$) was removed ($b = 0.50$, $t = 2.76$, $p = 0.007$). It seems that left-handedness is not predictive of sexual orientation in this sample, but 2D:4D ratio is.

A Californian Sample

The question of the relationship of 2D:4D to sexual orientation has also been considered in an excellent study by Marc Breedlove's group (see Williams et al. 2000). Their sample was 720 adults attending public street fairs in the San Francisco area. The participants consisted of 108 heterosexual and 277 homosexual men together with 146 heterosexual and 164 homosexual women. In the female sample the mean 2D:4D ratio of the right hand was significantly lower for homosexual women (0.96) compared to heterosexual women (0.97, $p = 0.03$). There were no differences between the mean 2D:4D of the left hand in lesbians (0.96) and heterosexual women (0.96). Homosexual women and heterosexual men had similar mean ratios in the right hand (0.96). Williams et al. (2000) concluded that lesbians had been exposed to high levels of prenatal androgens compared to heterosexual women. I think this conclusion is well founded, as Tortorice and Trivers have found a similar effect in a sample from New Jersey (personal communication).

The position regarding 2D:4D ratios in homosexual and heterosexual men was more complex. In the left hand homosexual men had higher mean 2D:4D (0.96) than heterosexuals (0.95) but the difference was not significant ($p = 0.09$). The homosexual and heterosexual mean 2D:4D ratios were very similar (0.95). There is no support here for different 2D:4D ratios and prenatal androgen concentrations in heterosexual and homosexual men. Nevertheless, there was an indication that homosexual men had substantially lower D_{r-l} than heterosexual men (Breedlove personal communication). This finding is consistent with the observation that D_{r-l} is low in left-handed subjects (Manning, Trivers et al. 2000). In addition, a consideration of number of older brothers in the male gay and heterosexual samples lead Williams et al. (2000) to suggest that homosexual men may be exposed to higher concentrations of prenatal androgens than heterosexuals. However, some caution needs to be used when interpreting data from gay street fairs. Attendance at these events is very high, and it is tempting to feel that such numbers give increased accuracy to the findings. Perhaps this is so, but one possible problem is that attendance is unlikely to be random in relation to 2D:4D ratio. For example, heterosexual women appear to substantially outnumber heterosexual men (Williams et al. 2000; Manning and Robinson unpublished data). There is therefore imbalance in representation relating to both gender and sexual orientation. Can we be confident that our samples of heterosexual men and women truly reflect the population norms for 2D:4D ratio? The mean 2D:4D ratios of homosexuals and heterosexuals recruited from street fairs should be confirmed from general population samples, which do not suffer from the self-selection problems inherent in voluntary attendance at gay events.

Fraternal Birth Order and Gay Men

Fraternal birth order is a widespread and robust correlate of male homosexuality. Gay men have a higher mean birth order than heterosexual men. This effect is associated with the number of older brothers. That is, the probability of homosexuality is dependent on the number of older brothers and is independent of the number of older sisters (Blanchard 1997; Blanchard and Bogaert 1996). The fraternal birth order effect may result from a maternal immune reaction, which is provoked by the male fetus but not by the female fetus. It has been suggested that the immune system is capable of "remembering" the number of male pregnancies but not the number of female pregnancies (Blanchard 1997). The result is, mothers alter their immune response to successive male babies. This proposed immune effect is not the only factor leading to homosexuality. Quantitative analysis suggests that only about one in seven gay men owe their sexual orientation to the influence of fraternal birth order.

The relationship of fraternal birth order to genetic influences on homosexuality is obscure. Nevertheless, the association between birth order and male homosexuality may relate to the expression of 2D:4D ratio. Suppose the immune response of mothers is to the testicular tissue of their sons. This may reduce the production of prenatal testosterone and compromise its organizational effect on the brain. If this is so, we should see an increase in the 2D:4D ratio of males (not necessarily gay males) with an increase in older brothers. On the other hand, it may be advantageous for later-born brothers to be exposed to high prenatal testosterone. This may increase their ability to compete against their older and larger male siblings. There is some evidence from birds that androgen concentrations may be increased in each subsequent egg of a clutch (Schwabl 1996). Presumably this enables small later-hatched chicks to compete in the nest with their larger brothers. Androgen levels of the egg can also be increased by mothers as a response to the attractiveness of their mate (Gil et al. 1999). In mammals it is more difficult to see how mothers could expose offspring to testosterone because aromatase would prevent movement of androgen across the placenta. However, it is possible that mothers may have some mechanism that influences fetal androgen levels (e.g., downregulation of placental aromatase). Alternatively, it may be possible that the male fetus increases testosterone production as a response to a physiological maternal trait that is correlated with the number of his older brothers. A possible example of such a trait may be the maternal immune response to successive sons. In summary, it is not clear whether testosterone concentrations would increase or decrease with subsequent male births.

An English Sample

In order to examine the relationships between 2D:4D and fraternal birth order Robinson and Manning (2000) recruited a sample of 285 men from northwest England. The participants were measured for 2nd and 4th digit length and their number of older brothers and sisters and younger brothers and sisters noted. There were 45 male homosexual subjects with Kinsey scores of greater than 3 in the sample. The remaining subjects were not questioned with regard to their sexual orientation, so that a few may have been gay. The homosexual men had a larger mean number of older siblings (1.75 ± 1.27 older sibs) than the heterosexual men (0.99 ± 1.66, $t = 3.45$, $p = 0.0006$). There was also a larger mean number of older brothers of homosexual men (0.98 ± 1.03 older brothers) compared to those for heterosexual men (0.52 ± 0.75 older brothers). There was no relationship between number of older brothers and 2D:4D ratio ($b = -0.001$, $F = 0.11$, $p = 0.74$). A simultaneous multiple regression with 2D:4D as the dependent variable and number of older brothers and sexual orientation (dummy coded heterosexual men = 1, homosexual men = 2) as the independent variable again showed no relationship between number of older brothers and 2D:4D ($b = 0.002$, $t = 0.64$, $p = 0.52$). However, there was a significant negative association between sexual orientation and 2D:4D, indicating again that 2D:4D was lower in gay men in comparison to heterosexual men. Adding number of older sisters, younger brothers, and younger sisters to the analysis revealed no new significant associations with 2D:4D ratio, but the association between sexual orientation and 2D:4D remained significant.

The relationship between 2D:4D ratio and fraternal birth order has been further tested by Manning (manuscript). Comparisons between 2D:4D ratio and birth order are influenced by variation in 2D:4D arising from within-family differences and between-family differences. We are interested in the former but not the latter. In order to remove between-family differences, 30 pairs of first- and second-born brothers were recruited. The 2nd and 4th digits of the left and right hand were measured and 2D:4D ratios calculated. There was little difference in the mean 2D:4D ratios of the right and left hands of first-born males (mean 2D:4D 0.976 ± 0.03) and second-born males (mean 2D:4D 0.973 ± 0.03). If on average the second-born brother had lower 2D:4D ratio than the first-born, then 2D:4D first-born minus 2D:4D second-born should be positive. However, there was no evidence of a significant difference in 2D:4D ratio in the right or left hand between brothers (mean 2D:4D ratio, older-younger brother = 0.001, $t = 0.12$, $p = 0.90$; right hand, older-younger brother = 0.008, $t = 1.2$, $p = 0.27$, left hand, older-younger brother = -0.005, $t = 0.51$, $p = 0.61$). These data indicate little support for a relationship between 2D:4D and fraternal birth order; however, they do not exclude the possibility of a weak association.

A Californian Sample

Marc Breedlove and his colleagues (Williams et al. 2000) have reported that men with a number of older male siblings have lower 2D:4D than men with few or no older brothers. In their sample of 385 men obtained from gay street fairs in San Francisco, they found that homosexual males had greater numbers of older brothers than heterosexual males. The 2D:4D ratio was lower for men with two or more older brothers compared to men without older brothers, and there was a significant negative correlation between the number of older brothers and 2D:4D of the right hand ($r = -0.10$, $p < 0.05$). In these data there is evidence that 2D:4D reduces with an increase in the numbers of older brothers. This is a further indication that mean 2D:4D is lower in homosexual men compared to heterosexual men. These data suggest that on average gay men are likely to have been exposed to higher androgen levels than heterosexual men.

Controls for Ethnicity

The 2D:4D ratios reported by Williams et al. (2000) show no significant difference between homosexual and heterosexual males. In fact if anything they indicate higher ratios in gay men. Why is this so? One possible confounding factor is that there is no control for ethnicity in their sample. This is not surprising because differences in 2D:4D between ethnic groups have only been very recently described (Manning, Barley et al. 2000). In a multiracial society these differences may affect the outcomes of 2D:4D studies, and obscure relationships between the ratio and variables other than ethnicity. Californian black college students have been shown to have 19% higher mean testosterone levels than white students and 21% higher concentrations of free testosterone (Ross et al. 1986). The differences were somewhat reduced by controlling for lifestyle factors, but overall they remained high and significant. It is likely that African Americans also have higher exposure to prenatal testosterone than Caucasian Americans, and therefore have lower 2D:4D than Caucasians. If this is so, an appreciable number of black subjects in the sample of Williams et al. (2000) may obscure differences between the sexes and between gay and heterosexual groups. The ethnic differences extend to subgroups within Caucasians (Manning, Barley et al. 2000), making it likely that populations, such as subjects of an Asian origin, may have different mean 2D:4D from European Caucasians. For example, a sample of 821 participants from England (Liverpool, $n = 403$), Southern India (Sugali and Yanadi Tribes, $n = 160$), and Natal (Zulu, $n = 258$) showed significant sex differences in mean 2D:4D ratio of the right hand (males 0.967 ± 0.04; females 0.972 ± 0.04, $t = 1.95$, $p = < 0.05$). There were also very significant differences in mean 2D:4D ratio for ethnicity (English 0.98 ± 0.04; Indian 0.97 ± 0.04; Zulu 0.95 ± 0.03; ANOVA $F = 61.81$, $p = 0.0001$). A two-factor ANOVA showed that the variance due to ethnicity was much greater than that due to sex (sex $F = 1.40$, $p = 0.24$; ethnicity $F = 61.16$, $p = 0.0001$; interaction $F = 1.27$, $p = 0.28$). The sample of Williams et al. (2000) shows low mean 2D:4D ratios varying from the highest of 0.97 for the right hand of heterosexual women down to 0.95 in the left hand of heterosexual men. It may be that the sample was a mix of ethnic groups.

Conclusions

I think the available data indicate the following: (a) homosexual women have lower 2D:4D ratios than heterosexuals, and this probably indicates the former are exposed to higher prenatal testosterone concentrations than the latter; (b) as for the men, there is some evidence that homosexuals have lower 2D:4D ratios than heterosexuals and that a correlate of male homosexuality, i.e., fraternal birth order, is also associated with homosexuality. However, surprisingly 2D:4D ratio appears to be correlated with Kinsey scores, so that exclusively homosexual men have higher values of 2D:4D ratios than men who are more ambivalent about their homosexuality. Bisexual men may therefore experience higher prenatal testosterone than exclusively homosexual men. More work is urgently needed to confirm and extend these associations. One way forward is to investigate the association between 2D:4D ratio and gender nonconformity, i.e., behavior somewhat like the opposite sex. Childhood gender nonconformity is the strongest correlate of adult sexual orientation (Bell et al. 1981; Bailey and Zucker 1995). However, not all homosexuals show childhood gender nonconformity. It would be of great interest to know whether a significant proportion of the variation in childhood gender nonconformity is predicted by 2D:4D ratio.

So where does this leave us in terms of the origin and maintenance of homosexuality? We do not yet understand the mechanism involved, and it is difficult to speculate on possible adaptive aspects of the phenotype. It may be that the action of sexually antagonistic genes can explain some of the variance in human sexual orientation. Such genes have different effects on fitness depending on which sex they are expressed in. Homosexuality reduces direct fitness, so that genes for high prenatal testosterone or high prenatal estrogen could have positive or negative effects depending on the sex of the individual they find themselves in. The overall fitness consequences of such genes depends on the sum of their effects in males and females. It is difficult or even impossible for such genes to be completely eliminated by natural selection. Another possibility is that homosexuality in some individuals may be the result of directional selection for higher prenatal concentrations of testosterone. Low 2D:4D in men may be associated with increased sperm counts, high prenatal and adult testosterone, greater lifetime reproductive success, good visual-spatial ability, and an efficient heart. Selection will be powerful for such male traits in groups where polygyny and or EPCs are common. High concentrations of testosterone may also have negative consequences on fitness, e.g., in predisposing toward autism and compromising verbal fluency. If female and male homosexuality is associated with high in utero androgen concentration this would be a further and very powerful factor that would oppose the spread of genes for high prenatal testosterone.

Alternatively homosexuality could be the result of genes that are associated with increases in indirect fitness through the action of kin selection (Hutchinson 1959; Weinrich 1987; Ruse 1981). In order to show that homosexuality is maintained by kin selection, it is necessary to demonstrate that by their actions gay men and women substantially increase the direct fitness of their heterosexual relatives. No such data are available.

So what is clear among this uncertainty? There are powerful biological influences on the etiology of an erotic attraction to same-sex partners. The hypothesis that homosexuality is an illness is untenable. Judging from patterns of 2D:4D the levels of in utero testosterone and estrogen may exert an effect on sexual orientation. Prenatal testosterone concentrations that are higher than normal may result in homosexuality in females. The etiology of male homosexuality and its relationship with 2D:4D is less certain, but both may show evidence of high prenatal testosterone. Bisexuality in males may be related to very high prenatal testosterone concentrations. These conclusions need to be further refined and tested across cultures and ethnic groups. One possibility is that genetic modifiers prevent homosexual orientation across much of the range of prenatal testosterone common to each group. The association of high testosterone and homosexuality needs to be viewed in the context of what is high for each geographical population or ethnic group. The actual mechanism underlying the effect of testosterone on sexual orientation is obscure. The expression of 2D:4D in gays and heterosexuals cannot help us in judging other theories, e.g., kin selection models, for the maintenance of homosexuality. We need more evidence on the mechanism that leads to a preference for same-sex partners, and what it is that is inherited. This knowledge will lead us to believable models for the maintenance of a trait that profoundly reduces direct fitness.

CHAPTER 8

Music, Musicians, and Mate Choice

Many human and nonhuman behaviors have no apparent survival value. Darwin (1871) pointed out that this is particularly so for traits associated with (a) courtship or (b) male:male competitive behavior for resources that may subsequently influence male access to females. The selective pressures acting on such behaviors have much to do with mating success and little to do with adaptation to the environment. Their maintenance is therefore thought to result from the action of sexual selection rather than natural selection (Darwin 1871). In this chapter I consider evidence for a correlation between 2D:4D and musical ability (a possible male courtship behavior). In chapter 9 I examine the relationship between 2D:4D ratio and a possible surrogate of male:male competition (competitive sport in general and the sport of football in particular).

Music as a Male Display Trait

Music requires time and energy in its production and has apparently no survival value in avoiding predation or in directly obtaining food. These are characteristics expected in courtship behaviors. This is not an idea original to me. Darwin (1871) himself argued in some detail that human music, along with bird song, had evolved as a result of sexual selection. Much work has been done on the sexual-selection aspects of bird song but little on human music as sexual courtship. The recent work of Miller (1998, 2000) and Miller and Todd (1995) is an exception to this trend. Miller (2000) has convincingly argued that similarities between human music, gibbon, whale, and bird song support a sexual-selection interpretation of music. Consistent with this he has shown successful human musicians are often male. Thus, a sample of 1,800 jazz albums, 1,500 rock albums, and over 3,800 classical works showed that for each genre there was a sex ratio of the principal music producers of 10:1 in favor of male musicians. In this sample male musical output peaked around age 30. Miller's sample includes the best music and musicians of each musical type. However, he points out that the sex bias in favor of males extends to all levels from local bands to prestigious concerts. This age- and sex-dependent pattern of musical productivity is exactly that predicted in any sexually selected trait. For example, Miller points out that Daly and Wilson (1994) have found similar age and sex patterns associated with human homicide. Of course, homicide is a repugnant crime. However, it probably represents the extreme expression of a great deal of violence that is often, but not always, directed toward young men by young men (Daly and Wilson 1994). Male:male violence is likely to be fashioned by intrasexual selection. Music may be the product of intersexual selection or mate choice.

Sluming and Manning (2000) have found similar evidence of a greater than expected male representation in symphony orchestras. The web sites of 18 symphony orchestras from Britain (5 orchestras), Continental Europe (9 orchestras), and North America (4 orchestras) showed men making up 60 to 97% of orchestras, with a mean of 80%. Although the general perception is that female representation is increasing, many of these orchestras have shown little change in their proportion of female musicians over the last 10 years.

Of course, music as sexual courtship does not mean that women are unable to appreciate or produce music. On the contrary, if musical ability is being used as a proxy for such traits as male fertility, women would need to be excellent judges of good music. Female performance in dichotic music listening tasks has been shown to be at least partly dependent on position in the menstrual cycle. Low estrogen concentrations are associated with a switch from interpretation by the left hemisphere to that of the right (Sanders and Wenmoth 1998). Ovulation is associated with a marked drop in estrogen concentrations. Therefore, periods of high fertility may be correlated with enhanced music appreciation.

Music and Fetal Conditions

Geschwind and Galaburda (1985a, 1985b, 1985c) have suggested that fetal testosterone may facilitate the growth of certain areas of the right hemisphere and thereby increase musical ability. There is some evidence to support this notion. Autism may be precipitated by high prenatal testosterone concentrations (Manning, Baron-Cohen et al. 2001). Autistic children, while profoundly handicapped in many of their cognitive processes, may show islets of high musical ability. Studies of blood flow in the brain of normal subjects suggest that there is right hemisphere lateralization for harmony perception in nonmusicians. Musicians may use both the right and left hemispheres for harmony perception, but it is not known whether this ability is congenital or the result of practice (Evers et al. 1999). Studies of patients with brain damage and cortectomy have also indicated an important role for the right hemisphere in the perception of pitch presented in isolation, in chords, and in melodies (Peretz 1990) and the discrimination of melodies by the use of contour and interval information (Liegeois-Chauvel 1998).

So is there a link between fetal testosterone production, sperm production, right hemisphere function, and musical ability? If there is, women could then use musical ability as an honest signal (i.e., a signal that males find difficult to fake) of male fertility. We have seen that there are associations between 2D:4D and sperm numbers and testosterone concentrations. Is 2D:4D ratio correlated with male musical ability?

2D:4D in Symphony Musicians

Sluming and Manning (2000) measured the 2D:4D ratio of 54 male and 16 female symphony musicians recruited from a major British symphony orchestra (the orchestra requested anonymity). The male musicians were from the following sections: violin (15 subjects), viola (6), cello (6), horn (6), bass (5), trombone (3), percussion (3), bassoon (3), clarinet (2), oboe (1), flute (1), trumpet (1), tuba (1), and timpani (1). The female sample included violin (5 subjects), viola (5), cello (2), harp (1), piccolo (1), oboe (1), and flute (1). For purposes of comparison controls were recruited (86 men and 78 women, ranging in age from 20 to 60 years) from adult social clubs and adult classes in the Merseyside area. Mean ages were similar in the musician groups (males, mean = 41.61 ± 10.19; females, mean = 33.00 ± 6.96 years) and in the control groups (males, mean = 41.83 ± 8.27 years; females, mean = 34.56 ± 7.75 years). The control catchment area included inner-city, suburban, and rural areas.

Male musicians had lower mean 2D:4D ratios in the left and right hand compared to controls (musicians, left hand 0.96 ± 0.03, right hand 0.93 ± 0.03; controls, left hand 0.98 ± 0.03, right hand 0.98 ± 0.04; see figure 8.1). The difference between mean 2D:4D ratios for musicians and controls was highly significant for both the left and right hands.

All the male musicians were Caucasian, but two were Scandinavian in origin. In view of the low 2D:4D ratios of Finnish males reported by Manning, Barley et al. (2000), these subjects were removed from the sample. The remaining sample of 52 musicians continued to show significantly lower 2D:4D than controls (left hand musicians 0.96 ± 0.03 and controls 0.98 ± 0.04, $t = 4.04$, $p = 0.0001$; right hand musicians 0.94 ± 0.03 and controls 0.98 ± 0.04, $t = 7.03$, $p = 0.0001$).

Female musicians had similar mean 2D:4D ratios to that of controls (means of right and left hands musicians, 0.99 ± 0.04; controls, 1.00 ± 0.04, $t - 0.57$, $p - 0.59$). Male and female musicians showed highly significant differences in mean 2D:4D; i.e., males had lower 2D:4D than

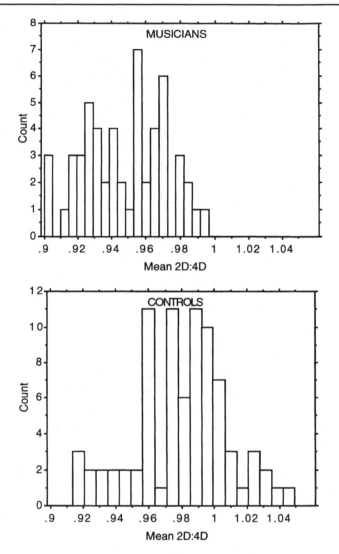

Figure 8.1. The distribution of the mean 2D:4D ratio of the left and right hand of 54 male symphony musicians and 86 male controls. The male musicians have lower 2D:4D ratios than controls (independent samples t test, right hand, $t = 7.34$, $p = 0.0001$ Bonferroni adjustment $p = 0.0002$; left hand, $t = 4.32$, $p = 0.0001$).

females ($t = 5.27$, $p = 0.0001$). It is therefore inappropriate that male and female samples should be pooled.

The data suggest that it is unlikely that low digit ratio helps with the actual mechanics of playing. Different instrument groups showed no evidence of different mean ratios; for example, for men, strings $n = 23$, left hand 0.96 ± 0.03, nonstrings $n = 31$, 0.96 ± 0.03, $t = 0.45$, $p = 0.65$; right

hand strings 0.93 ± 0.03, nonstrings 0.94 ± 0.03, $t = 0.57$, $p = 0.57$. Similarly in women there were no significant differences between the ratios of
string and nonstring players. A relatively long 4th digit compared to the
length of the 2nd does not appear to facilitate the mechanics of playing
particular instruments.

Within instrument groups symphony musicians are ranked in a highly
hierarchical way. In the largest group, the male violinists, there was evidence that the musicians rated most highly by their colleagues had the
lowest 2D:4D ratios (see figure 8.2).

Considering the sections with two or more male musicians, the participants were divided into two groups. One contained the top-ranked musician down to the middle-ranked, the other consisted of the lower-ranked
subjects. There were 20 subjects in the former and 19 in the latter group.
The mean 2D:4D ratio of the left hand was significantly lower in the high-
ranked group ($n = 20$, 0.95 ± 0.03) compared to the lower-ranked musicians ($n = 19$, 0.97 ± 0.02, $t = 3.15$, $p = 0.003$, adjustment for multiple
tests $p = 0.006$). A similar but weaker and nonsignificant difference was
found for the right hand (high-ranked 0.92 ± 0.03; low-ranked 0.94 ±
0.02, $t = 1.46$, $p = 0.15$).

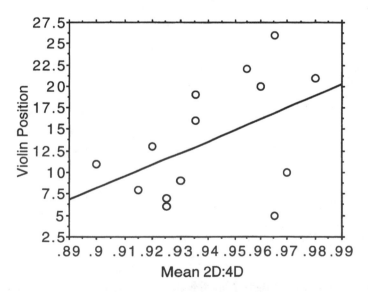

Figure 8.2. The relationship between mean 2D:4D ratio of the left and right hands of 14
male violinists and their hierarchical position within the violin section of a major symphony orchestra. Low values on the violin position axis indicate high rank within the
section. Musicians with low 2D:4D ratio ranked higher than musicians with high 2D:4D
ratio (left hand, $b = 208.61$, $F = 7.10$, $p = 0.02$ Bonferroni adjustment $p = 0.04$; right
hand $b = 68.67$, $F = 1.45$, $p = 0.25$).

The position of a musician within the hierarchy of an orchestra is ostensibly judged by perceptions of their musical ability by their colleagues within the section, and to a lesser extent, by other members of the orchestra. Within any male hierarchy there is likely to be an effect on rank of assertiveness and aggression. It is not possible to say with certainty that rank within the orchestra is determined primarily by musical ability (which is the position accepted within the orchestra) or by testosterone-mediated competitiveness. The latter may, for example, increase drive and lead to an increase in practice time and therefore perceived musical ability. However, it is persuasive that Geschwind and Galaburda's hypothesis of testosterone-mediated effects on musical ability has led to a prediction that low 2D:4D ratio would be related to entry and rank within a symphony orchestra and that this has been supported by the data. It seems likely that innate musical ability is an important component in the makeup of musicians who eventually attain the standard necessary to play at the very highest levels. Further work should now be done, e.g., in relating tests of musical ability per se to 2D:4D ratio and correlating 2D:4D ratio with rankings of individual musicians across orchestras. This work will have to be done carefully because in the final analysis the judgment of what is very good music as opposed to merely good music is subjective.

Can 2D:4D ratio be used in the identification and encouragement of talented musicians early in their development? This depends how accurately one can predict the development of musical talent in young people using conventional methods, and how much more accurate this process would be if it were informed by the use of 2D:4D. It is certainly not appropriate to simply select boys with low 2D:4D ratio and expect them all to show high musical ability as children and adults. However, within groups of already talented young musicians, their 2D:4D ratio, because it shows little change at puberty, may help to identify those who will develop further into highly talented musicians. An inspection of data shows that the mean 2D:4D ratio of a sample of elite violinists correlates with their position within a symphony orchestra (see figure 8.2). In fact the 2D:4D ratio predicts 22% of the variance of orchestral position. Because musical ability is a matter of opinion, we do not know whether position in the orchestra is indeed a valid measure, and of course it may itself be affected by such factors as age. That is, as members of the orchestra age, they may wish to change their position so that they are asked to be involved in less-demanding pieces of music. If age is an important factor in determining orchestral position, it will tend to weaken the relationship between 2D:4D and musical ability. The 2D:4D ratio may be more closely associated with musical ability than the relationship between 2D:4D and orchestral position suggests. On the other hand it may be that orchestral position is related to male competitiveness as discussed above. In this case 2D:4D may have less predictive power in relation to musical ability than the association in the data suggests. The matter can only be resolved by longitudinal studies that test changes in ability in young musicians over a period of a number of years.

This study may be the first quantitative attempt to investigate the association between 2nd and 4th digit length and musical ability. It is legitimate to ask whether nonscientists have noticed such an association. In the musician sample all of the participants had longer 4th digits than 2nd, and the differences in some subjects were greater than 1 cm. It is likely that such asymmetries in the same hand are noticeable to even a casual observer. Sorell (1968) pointed out that musical ability has been linked with very long ring fingers for many years. He illustrated this with handprints from composers such as Alexander Tcherepnin and Edgar Varese, but the most powerful image he showed in this context was that of a cast of Franz Liszt's right hand (Sorell 1968, 187). In this cast Liszt's ring finger is strikingly dominant in length, with the middle phalanx making up an apparently disproportionate part of the finger. These are anecdotal observations, but measurements of casts and photographs of the hands of eminent musicians may well reveal very low 2D:4D ratios.

Music and Female Choice

The data from the study of 2D:4D in a symphony orchestra indicate that elite male musicians have lower 2D:4D ratios than the population norm. They also suggest that within the elite group there are hierarchical differences that support a relationship between musical ability and low 2D:4D ratio. What of evidence that women are using musical ability in their judgments of attractiveness? Common-sense observations of the interest shown by females in popular musicians are consistent with a sexual selection payoff for gifted musicians. For example, Miller (2000) discusses the lifestyle of successful popular male musicians and their female "groupies." He concludes that there is much anecdotal evidence that male musicians are perceived as sexually attractive by women. There is probably some truth in these observations because they are consistent with popular perceptions, but it is important to make this kind of enquiry as quantitative as possible. Sluming and Manning (2000) reported observations of the sex composition of audiences in seats that were close and seats at some distance from the orchestra. In their observations of 11 symphony concerts, they found evidence that women tended to be present in higher than expected numbers in the front stalls. In total, 1,750 members of the audience were counted. In the first four rows of the center stalls there was a total of 820

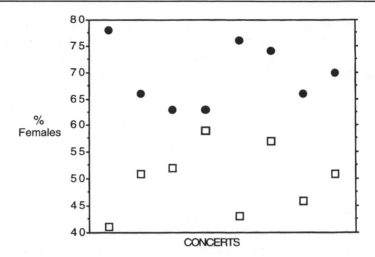

Figure 8.3. In a sample of 11 symphony concerts women tended to be more frequently represented in the first four rows of the stalls (solid symbols, an average of 69% women) during concerts than men. There was no excess of females (open symbols, an average of 51% women) or males in the back rows. The difference between the representation of women in the front and back stalls was significant ($X^2 - 56.47$, $p = 0.0001$).

individuals made up of 69% women and 31% men. In the last four rows there were 930 individuals with 51% women and 49% men. In all concerts there was a greater percentage of women in the front stalls compared to the back (see figure 8.3).

The finding that women are more frequently represented than men in seats close to the orchestra may be interpreted in a number of different ways. For example, front-stall seats are often less expensive than back-stall seats, and this may correlate with the socioeconomic status of the audience at the front. Maybe this relates in some way to the sex composition of these groups also. In this sample some of these concerts had this price differential and others did not. The sex ratio was not noticeably different when seats were less expensive at the front compared to when they were the same price as the rest of the stalls.

I do not place emphasis on these observations but offer them as an example of how the sexual selection theory of music may be tested. Further work could, for example, look at the age composition of the audience in addition to their sex. Also if concerts are pay-at-the-door, the position in the cycle of premenopausal women may relate to their seating positions relative to the orchestra. Further empirical testing of the courtship theory of music is now highly desirable.

Darwin (1871) pointed to the universality of music in human groups and, through time, how music arouses strong emotions and how the lyrics of songs are very often concerned with love. He concluded that musical tones and rhythm were used by our ancestors during courtship and that music itself may have preceded speech. This is not to say that musicians when they perform do so with a sexual motive in mind. As Darwin points out, the "impassioned orator, bard, or musician" may not suspect that he is using the same means by which his "ancestors long ago aroused each other's ardent passions, during their courtship and rivalry."

Miller (2000) has taken up these arguments. He suggests that there are a number of criteria that music fulfills which indicate it is a biological adaptation: (a) it is universal across cultures and recorded history; (b) it shows a predictable developmental pattern in individuals, resulting in musical capacity in all normal humans relative to closely related species; (c) almost everyone can learn a melody, carry a tune, and appreciate musical performances; (d) it involves specialized memory capacity so that adults can reproduce thousands of melodies; (e) musical abilities show cortical lateralization and are found in specialized cortical areas; (f) there are similarities between human music and "song" in birds, gibbons, and whales; and (g) music is capable of stimulating intense emotion, suggesting adaptation for perception in addition to production of music.

Despite this circumstantial evidence that music is an adaptation, it is difficult to see how it can increase nonsexually selected components of fitness such as survivorship. It may be that music is a group adaptation. It is often performed by groups of musicians for large audiences. It could function to reinforce a perception of a group identity. However, group selection is a weak force. It may have been important in the evolution and maintenance of sex because sexual populations accumulate beneficial mutations faster than asexuals (Manning and Thompson 1984). However, this example aside, group selection is unlikely to have been powerful enough to encourage the spread of musical ability.

Reliability and Signals of Mate Quality

Females will evolve to respond to male signals of fertility if the signals are reliable, i.e., if they are difficult for males to fake. The concept of reliable signals raises practical and theoretical questions.

Cost and Reliability of Signals

There are probably a number of signals that are correlated with such traits as fertility and genetic variation in fitness. In the past it has been challenged whether genetic variation in fitness is high. This is because theorists have assumed that selection will eliminate genes that negatively affect longevity, fertility, etc. The heritability of fitness was therefore said to be close to zero. More recently the additive genetic coefficient of variation (Cv_a, the genetic standard deviation of a trait, standardized by the trait mean and multiplied by 100) has been used to estimate genetic variation in fitness (Houle 1992). It turns out that in humans and other animals fitness-related traits often have higher values of Cv_a than morphological traits (e.g., human fecundity has a Cv_a of 15 to 20 which is four to five times greater than that of height; Burt 1995). So it is possible that potential mates display signals of fertility and even "good genes." Such signals, if they are not costly, may be mimicked by genes that "cheat," hence the concept of mate choice for traits that involve a cost or exert a handicap on the displaying individual (Zahavi 1975, 1977).

An example of a "costly" trait associated with human mate choice is fluctuating asymmetry. Humans and many other animals are bilaterally symmetrical. This means that the growth trajectory of the right and left sides is designed to maintain symmetry during periods of growth and to ensure that when growth stops the adult is symmetrical. Most individuals do not show perfect symmetry in all paired traits such as ear size, finger length, wrist thickness, etc. These small, random deviations from symmetry are FA. Symmetry in humans is probably energetically expensive to maintain during periods of rapid growth (Wilson and Manning 1996), and sexually selected traits such as breasts may show high levels of asymmetry (Møller et al. 1995; Manning et al. 1996). There is evidence of mate choice for symmetry in humans. In comparison with asymmetrical men, symmetrical men report more sexual partners (Thornhill and Gangestad 1994; Waynforth 1998), more extra-pair sexual partners (Gangestad and Thornhill 1997), and more children (Waynforth 1998). They are also rated as more attractive (Grammer and Thornhill 1994) and may stimulate more orgasms in their sexual partners than asymmetrical men (Thornhill et al. 1995).

Music as a Costly Signal

Prenatal testosterone concentrations are likely to be dependent on the level of function of the fetal testes, including potential for sperm production. If testosterone facilitates right hemisphere function, females may be sensitive to any evidence of this in males. Musical ability is probably such a signal. Yes, performance with a musical instrument can be improved with practice, but very high performance levels are not likely to be attained by practice alone. Innate musical ability may well correlate with fertility. Women who prefer men with musical ability may have sons who also show the phenotype of high fertility and musicality. Such sons would be likely to make many grandchildren. The genes for a sexual preference for musical ability and the trait of musical ability would therefore tend to spread together and to become closely linked on the same chromosome. In such a system, as choosy females become more common, the payoff to musical males increases. This is Fisher's theory of runaway selection (Fisher 1930).

Runaway selection is not a powerful process when the genes for female preference and the male display trait are costly and present in low frequency. Once the choice and display genes become more common, the runaway process is a powerful one leading to an elaboration of the male trait. If the runaway process is all that is operating, then the display trait will have no payoff to females in the fitness of their male offspring other than their attractiveness to females with the choice gene. Fisher's process may be important in the evolution of human musical ability. For example, Miller (2000) suggests that the runaway process favors the evolution of more and more complex male acoustic signals. However, I think female choice genes for male musical ability were first favored because musical ability identified men with high sperm counts and high sperm quality. Male fertility is an immediate benefit to females, which may or may not be related to the difficult question of whether females choose males with "good genes." Of course this first stage is now gone and directional selection has left its mark in the form of the elaborated trait of musical ability. I guess this means we must thank female choice for the gift of human music. Whether high musical ability indicates only fertility in males or both fertility and good genes is a question that must be resolved. It may be investigated by relating 2D:4D ratio to many fitness domains such as fertility, physiological and cognitive efficiency, and survivorship.

Conclusions

Patterns of 2D:4D may help to settle arguments relating to sexual selection in humans. One such issue is the origin and function of human music. Darwin (1871) and more recently Miller (1998, 2000) and Miller and Todd (1995) have suggested that music is essentially associated with courtship and has been elaborated by the action of female choice. Evidence from the pattern of male 2D:4D in a symphony orchestra compared to population controls, and within the orchestra in relation to perceived musical ability, is supportive of the notion of music as a male display trait. Low 2D:4D may correlate with both musical ability and fertility.

CHAPTER 9

Sporting Ability, Running Speed, Spatial Perception, Football Players, and Male Competition

In this chapter I explore whether 2D:4D ratio is a correlate of human sporting ability. Particular attention is given to football (soccer) and running, but the arguments may be generalizable to many sports. Competitive human sport is characterized by actions that recall male:male fighting. Kicking, throwing, and punching are all actions commonplace in sport. Boxing, contact martial arts, and fencing involve striking opponents. In other sports these actions are directed at objects such as balls and pucks. However, in essence there are similarities between skills shown in soccer, American football, cricket, baseball, tennis, et cetera, and skills used in fighting. Often sporting skills are demonstrations of visual-spatial abilities. In addition many sports demand high levels of pace and endurance. High prenatal testosterone concentrations may be an essential precursor for excellence in such activities.

As with music, males predominate as participants in sport. However, unlike music, sport may often be a male spectator activity. Thus sporting ability does not appear to be a male display trait. Rather, sport may act as a proxy for direct male:male combat. Rivalry is intense and often acrimonious in sporting activity. Contestants compete within boundaries established by rules, but the limits of such rules are repeatedly tested in every contest. Contests must be strongly policed by officials who have absolute control of conduct. There is always the possibility that the contest will change from a highly structured sporting activity to a fight. Male spectators often align themselves with one contestant or one team. Rivalry between groups of spectators is also intense, often leading to fighting. Success at the highest levels in sport is rewarded with great status and often with large sums of money. Men who accumulate status and financial rewards from sport are likely to prove attractive to women. Thus sport has many of the characteristics of one component of sexual selection, i.e., male:male competition for resources that lead to the acquisition of females (Darwin 1871). Of course, if this argument is correct, it does not exclude the possibility that women may choose sportsmen because success in sport is directly related to traits such as fertility. Visual-spatial ability and vascular efficiency may be associated with high sperm counts and prenatal testosterone concentrations. Women may obtain high fertility, status, and resources from successful sportsmen.

2D:4D and Sporting Ability

There may be systematic differences in 2D:4D ratio between participants of different sports. I do not address this question. Instead, I first ask whether sporting ability is negatively related to 2D:4D independent of type of sport.

2D:4D and Ability across Many Sports

Manning and Taylor (2001) have examined the relationship between 2D:4D and rank in a range of sports. In this study there were 128 male participants with a mean age of 22.35 ± 4.91 years. Subjects were recruited on a university campus, and most were students and staff. A questionnaire was used to establish the sporting rank of participants (see table 9.1). Subjects were asked to select their most suitable rank for their favorite sport. This questionnaire was first used by Manning and Pickup (1998) in assessments of performance of middle-distance runners. The rankings derived from the questionnaire were significantly correlated with best running times for 800 meters and 1,500 meters in the Manning and Pickup (1998) study.

The 128 participants had a mean 2D:4D ratio of 0.98 ± 0.03 for both right and left hands. This was very similar to population norms for Merseyside and suggested the sample was not biased for extremes of 2D:4D. The subjects practiced seven sports (running 45% of participants,

Table 9.1. Sports performance questionnaire

Please choose your most suitable rank for your sporting activity. Start from rank 10 and work down.

Rank	Criteria
10.	You have represented your country
9.	You think you could represent your country
8.	You have competed at national level
7.	You think you could compete at national level
6.	You have competed at county level
5.	You think you could compete at county level
4.	You have competed at an organized level
3.	You think you can compete at an organized level
2.	Your sport is only social
1.	You do no sport

Table 9.2. 2D:4D ratio as a predictor of high sporting rank

Trait	β	t	p
2D:4D right	6.18	4.22	0.0001
Age	0.07	2.03	0.04
Experience	−0.03	0.76	0.45
Type of sport	−0.09	1.11	0.27

football 14%, martial arts 10%, rugby 8%, tennis or squash 8%, swimming 7%, hockey 5%) to various levels of ability. There were 3 participants (2%) who engaged in no sports. The mean rank of sporting achievement of the sample was 5.33 ± 2.01, and the mean experience at their sport 5.33 ± 4.44 years.

The 2D:4D ratio of the right hand was a significant predictor of sporting rank, with low 2D:4D associated with high rank ($b = -25.87$, $F = 17.40$, $p = 0.0001$, Bonferroni adjusted $p = 0.0002$). The 2D:4D ratio of the left hand was also negatively related to sporting rank, but the association was just outside significance ($b = -12.19$, $F = 3.75$, $p = 0.055$). Subjects with lower 2D:4D in the right hand compared to the left had higher rank than those with right ratio higher than left (rank regressed on D_{r-l}, $b = -17.87$, $F = 5.45$, $p = 0.02$).

Sporting rank is likely to be influenced by age and experience. It may also be easier to attain high rank in those sports practiced by few participants. A simultaneous multiple regression analysis showed that 2D:4D of the right hand remained a significant predictor of sporting rank after the effect of age, experience, and type of sport were removed (see table 9.2). As expected, the older subjects had attained higher rank than the younger. Presumably this reflects more opportunity to move up the rankings.

2D:4D and Visual-Spatial Judgment in Men

It is likely that many sports test visual-spatial judgment. Striking a moving opponent or ball requires fine judgment of distance. Determining the exact point of impact demands an accurate perception of the surface of the target as it moves through space, in addition to an awareness of the relative movement of one's own hand, foot, head, and so forth. Geschwind and Galaburda (1985a, 1985b, 1985c) suggested that prenatal testosterone enhances the growth of the right hemisphere and is, as a consequence, associated with good spatial abilities. Is the 2D:4D ratio a predictor of spatial skills?

Visual-spatial abilities were tested in a subset (78 subjects) of the sample using the Judgment of Line Orientation Test (JLOT) and the Vandenberg

Mental Rotations Test (MRT). Men perform better on average than women in both these tests, but the MRT shows more marked sexual dimorphism in the scores. In the JLOT subjects were shown a drawing of a vertically orientated vessel containing liquid. The surface of the liquid was marked by a horizontal line. Subjects were asked to draw a line representing the surface of liquid in a tilted container. The line should of course be horizontal. Angular deviations from the horizontal are used as a negative index of performance in the test. In the sample of 78 men, the mean angle of deviation was 2.90 ± 2.60 degrees. The prediction was that high 2D:4D ratio would be associated with high angular deviation. Positive associations were in fact found, but they were not significant (right hand $b = 3.36$, $F = 0.07$, $p = 0.80$; left hand $b = 16.49$, $F = 1.96$, $p = 0.17$).

The MRT shows higher differences between men and women than the JLOT. The version of the MRT used in this instance contained 20 items, and the time limit was 10 minutes. Each item consisted of a criterion figure, two correct alternatives, and two incorrect. The correct alternatives were identical to the criterion figure but were drawn in a rotated position. The distracters were rotated mirror images of the criterion figure in half the items while the other items contained distracters that were rotated images of one or two of the other structures. Two points were given for a line that was correct for both choices; none for a line in which one was correct or both incorrect. If only one figure was chosen and it was correct then one point was given. This system of marking eliminates the need to apply a correction for guessing. Our prediction was that low 2D:4D ratio would be associated with high MRT scores. There was, in fact, a negative relationship for both right and left hands (right hand 2D:4D $b = -63.91$, $F = 10.87$, $p = 0.002$; left hand 2D:4D $b = -74.31$, $F = 19.33$, $p = 0.0001$, adjusted for multiple tests $p = 0.0002$).

This study supports the position that low 2D:4D is predictive of high sporting potential and good spatial ability in men. The relationship appears to be robust over a number of sports. Exposure to high concentrations of prenatal testosterone may well influence the central nervous system and perhaps other organ systems. The result is an increase in the abilities necessary for effective male:male competition.

2D:4D and Running Speed

Is 2D:4D ratio a strong predictor of performance among participants of a sport? We can best answer this question in those sports where performance is readily measured and where it is not mainly a question of opinion.

Running, with its reliance and emphasis on accurate times, is one such discipline. Manning and Vella (manuscript) have examined 2D:4D and running speed in men who regularly train for and compete in 800 m and 1,500 m races. The participants were 71 young men (mean age 22.93 ± 2.03 years) who at the time of measurement trained on average 2.5 times per week and who had run in timed middle-distance races. Performance was measured by taking the mean time of the athlete's last three races. This was available for 47 participants in 800 m races and for 40 participants in 1,500 m races. The runners were recruited from athletics clubs in Liverpool and London, and the mean 2D:4D ratio of the right and left hand of participants (0.98 ± 0.03) was similar to that reported for a large sample of Liverpool men (Manning et al. 1998). Mean times were 143.09 ± 16.80 seconds for the 800 m and 258.97 ± 19.64 seconds for the 1,500 m, and the lowest mean times in the sample (113.25 seconds for the 800 m and 227.97 seconds for the 1,500 m) suggested the fastest runners were of regional or county standard.

Men with low 2D:4D ratio reported faster times than men with high 2D:4D ratio for 800 m and 1,500 m (1,500 m right $b = 305.90$, $F = 11.94$, $p = 0.001$, Bonferroni correction $p = 0.002$; left $b = 850.07$, $F = 0.79$, $p = 0.38$; 800 m see figure 9.1). Other variables, including weight, height, training frequency per week, systolic and diastolic blood pressure, and pulse rate, did not predict running speed. Age was a weak predictor of 800 m times; older subjects tended to report faster times than younger athletes

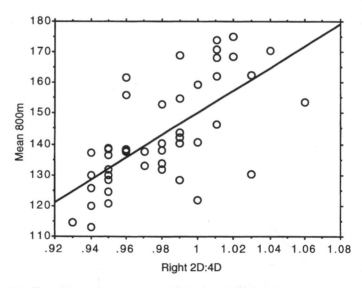

Figure 9.1. The relationship between 2D:4D of the right hand of 47 male athletes and the mean of their last three 800 meters times (right hand $b = 361.49$, $F = 36.45$, $p = 0.0001$, Bonferonni correction $p = 0.0002$; left hand $b = 127.31$, $F = 3.92$, $p = 0.05$). Subjects with low 2D:4D ratios recorded faster times than athletes with high 2D:4D ratios.

($b = -2.62$, $F = 4.27$, $p = 0.04$), but not of 1,500 m times. This was presumably the result of the cumulative effect of years of training. When the influence of age was removed, right 2D:4D remained a significant predictor of running speed (simultaneous multiple regression test: 800 m right 2D:4D $b = 344.03$, $t = 5.18$, $p = 0.001$, Bonferonni correction $p = 0.0002$; 1,500 m right 2D:4D $b = 295.06$, $t = 3.06$, $p = 0.004$).

The 2D:4D of the right hand was a better predictor of running speed than the 2D:4D of the left. The former predicted 38% of the variance in running speed in the 800 m and 30% of the running speed in the 1,500 m. The latter predicted only 7% of the variance in speed for the 800 m and 1% of the variance in the 1,500 m. Athletes who had lower 2D:4D ratios in the right hand compared to the left ran faster than those with ratios that were lower in the left than the right (times regressed on D_{r-l}: 800 m $b = 279.56$, $F = 4.39$, $p = 0.04$; 1,500 m $b = 512.51$, $F = 9.43$, $p = 0.004$).

Does this result mean that 2D:4D can be used to select young runners with high potential? The performance of prepubertal or pubertal athletes may not correlate well with eventual best performance as an adult because of variation in developmental rates. It is likely that the variation in 2D:4D within groups of young runners can be used as a predictor of adult running performance, which can be used in addition to other predictors. The way to confirm this is through careful longitudinal studies of 2D:4D and running speed across puberty.

2D:4D and Cross-Cultural Tests of Mental Rotation

The study of sport and 2D:4D ratio revealed unexpectedly strong relationships between 2D:4D ratio and MRT. Is this association general for men, and is it found in women also? I now discuss data on 2D:4D ratio and MRT from samples of men and women obtained from Liverpool and Hungary and a composite sample from London and Sweden (Sanders, Bereczkei, Csatho, and Manning, manuscript).

There were 47 men and 51 women in the Liverpool sample, 44 men and 44 women Hungarian participants, and 24 men and 24 women in the sample from London and Sweden. As expected the mean MRT scores were consistently and significantly higher for men compared to women in all three samples (Liverpool mean MRT, men $= 24.61 \pm 8.88$ and women $= 16.98 \pm 8.68$; Hungary men $= 22.25 \pm 7.24$ and women $= 11.93 \pm 5.01$; London/Sweden men $= 22.17 \pm 3.10$ and women $= 15.88 \pm 4.22$).

Our prediction for men was that low 2D:4D ratios would be associated with good spatial skills, i.e., high MRT scores. We therefore used one-tailed tests. In women the expectation was less clear and two-tailed tests were used. I consider here the relationships between mean 2D:4D of the right and left hands and MRT scores. In the Liverpool sample 2D:4D ratio was a significant negative predictor of MRT scores in males; i.e., men with low 2D:4D excelled at the MRT ($b = -64.06$, $F = 5.29$, $p = 0.01$ one-tailed, adjusted for multiple tests $p = 0.03$). In women there was a positive but nonsignificant relationship ($b = 56.38$, $F = 1.64$, $p = 0.21$). The Hungarian sample also showed a negative and significant relationship between 2D:4D and MRT in men ($b = -12.49$, $F = 4.69$, $p = 0.02$ one-tailed adjusted for multiple tests $p = 0.04$). There was a weak negative association in females, but this was not significant ($b = -2.41$, $F = 0.73$, $p = 0.40$). The sample from London and Sweden was small (24 men and 24 women). Nevertheless, men with low 2D:4D ratio had higher MRT scores than men with high 2D:4D ($b = -5.08$, $F = 3.93$, $p = 0.03$ one-tailed). There was a very weak and nonsignificant negative association in women ($b = -0.59$, $F = 0.01$, $p = 0.91$). The relationships between 2D:4D and MRT score in the pooled sample of men ($n = 115$) and women ($n = 119$) are shown in figure 9.2. There was a significant negative association between 2D:4D and MRT in the male sample, but the slope of the line in the female sample was close to zero.

Lower 2D:4D ratios in the right hand compared to the left did not appear to be an important predictor of MRT in these data. The Liverpool sample did show that men with low values of D_{r-l} had high MRT scores ($b = -9.33$, $F = 4.19$, $p = 0.027$ one-tailed). There was no evidence of this pattern in the other samples.

These data are further support for an association of high MRT scores with low 2D:4D or malelike ratios. However, male:male competition is likely to involve a range of abilities. Individuals that excel at sports may have most of these abilities, but some sports are more likely to test a greater range of traits than others.

2D:4D and Football

Football, or soccer, is a game that tests many of the characteristics which may be reasonably associated with success in male:male fighting. It is played by two teams each of 11 participants (usually males, although organized female soccer is gaining popularity). The main action is that of kicking a ball, but the ball may also be struck with the head. Fine judgment is possible in kicking. The player may weight the strike in order to control the distance, or he may kick the ball asymmetrically so that it "bends" in the air. The teams attempt to kick the ball into a rectangular space bounded by wooden posts, i.e., their opponent's goal. The goal is guarded by a keeper who is the only player allowed to handle the ball. He

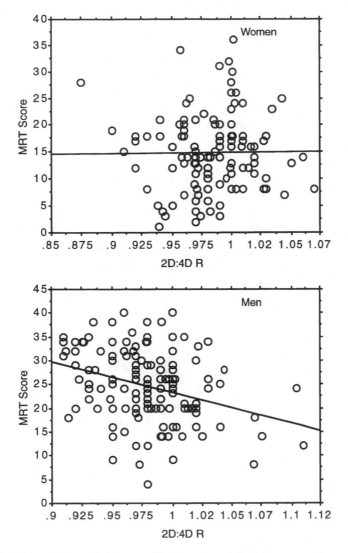

Figure 9.2. The relationship between 2D:4D and mental rotation scores (a measure of spatial perception) in men and women from Liverpool, Hungary, and a sample obtained from London and Sweden (right hand $b = -64.72$, $F = 16.52$, $p = 0.0001$ Bonferroni correction $p = 0.0002$; left hand $b = -31.07$, $F = 3.94$, $p = 0.05$). Men with low right-hand 2D:4D ratios or male-type ratios scored higher on the Mental Rotation Test than men with high 2D:4D ratios or female-type ratios. This relationship remained significant after population differences were removed ($b = -60.13$, $t = 4.02$, $p = 0.0001$). There was no consistent trend in the female sample ($b = 2.32$, $F = 0.01$, $p = 0.91$).

may also kick or punch the ball in his attempts to keep it from entering the goal. In professional leagues or competitions, football is played at great speed and pace, and in most games endurance and skills are tested to the utmost. At elite levels all players have great skill, and very small differences in ability are accentuated and recognized through repeated testing over many games. This is the "beautiful game" that draws many thousands of spectators. Its elite exponents are rewarded by high status and wealth.

2D:4D in Professional Football Players

Football tests visual-spatial abilities in directing the ball at the goal and at teammates. Pace and endurance are also tested. Football players are likely to have low 2D:4D ratios, i.e., to have experienced high testosterone and low estrogen levels in utero. Furthermore, accomplished football players are likely to have lower 2D:4D ratios than less-gifted players. These predictions have been examined by Manning and Taylor (2001).

Football began in England, but is now popular throughout the world. In England professional football clubs compete within four leagues or competitions. In decreasing order of excellence they are: the Premier Division, the 1st Division, the 2nd Division, and the lowest, the 3rd Division. At the end of each season the bottom clubs in each league are relegated to the league below and replaced by the top clubs of the lower divisions. The bottom club of the third is relegated to nonleague football. The league position of clubs is the focus of intense competition, and the Premiership and 1st Division are the usual competitions in which one finds established and accomplished players.

Each club has a squad of 15 to 20 players from which the first team is regularly chosen. Reserves are also employed. They cover for first-team players in the event of injury. Often two youth teams are maintained in which players are generally in the age range of 16 to 18 years. If judged good enough, players may progress from the youth teams to the first-team squad. Clubs do not obtain all their players from their youth teams. Many highly accomplished players are transferred from club to club in exchange for large sums of money.

The Sample

We measured 2D:4D ratios in the season 1998–1999 from players in the following clubs: Premier League, Liverpool and Coventry; 1st Division, Sunderland and Tranmere; 2nd Division, Preston and Oldham; and 3rd Division, Cambridge and Rochdale. The numbers of participants per division were Premiership, 48; 1st Division, 62; 2nd Division, 77; 3rd Division, 68. Many of the better players go on to become coaches. The staff of the clubs in the sample provided 21 of these well-known ex-players. In addition, in order to obtain participants of the very highest ability, we measured 30 players who, during the celebrations of the 100th anniversary of the Football League, were judged to be in the top 100 best players of that period. These very high status men played in the period between 1936 and 1999. Most were of home nation origin (England, Scotland, Wales, Northern Ireland, and Eire) and the mean number of appearances or "caps" for their country was 48.17 ± 33.44 with a range from 1 to 125. Their names together with the English clubs they played for are provided in table 9.3.

There were 305 professional football players in the sample. In addition 533 controls were recruited from Merseyside males between the ages of 17 to 41 years. The total sample was 839 men.

Patterns of 2D:4D in Professional Football Players and Controls

The professional football players tended to have lower 2D:4D ratios (mean 0.95 ± 0.03) than controls (mean 0.98 ± 0.04, $t = 14.78$, $p = 0.0001$; see figure 9.3). The mean 2D:4D for men in the Merseyside area is 0.98. In comparison our control sample consisted of 50% of men with 2D:4D less than 0.98, while the sample of players had 90% of its number with less than 0.98. This illustrates the preponderance of extreme male-type ratios in the sample of players.

The associations were similar for right and left hands. For brevity I give details for 2D:4D of the left hand. Within the sample of players there were significant variations in 2D:4D ratio. The elite "stars" had a mean 2D:4D in the left hand of 0.94, as did the coaches. Within the leagues, the Premier Division players had a mean of 0.95, 1st Division 0.94, 2nd Division 0.95, and 3rd Division 0.95. The control mean showed a large increase to 0.98. These between-group differences were highly significant (ANOVA, $F = 37.31$, $p = 0.0001$). Ranking the groups on probable overall "football ability" (stars = -2, coaches = -1, premier players = 0, and 1st, 2nd, and 3rd Divisions as 1, 2 and 3, and Controls as 4) showed that 2D:4D ratio was a significant negative predictor of position within this ranking ($b = 0.009$, $F = 163.02$, $p = 0.0001$; see figure 9.4). Considering the players and ex-players only, there was a significant increase in 2D:4D ratio from the "stars" to the players in the 3rd Division ($b = 0.002$, $F = 4.12$, $p = 0.04$). This suggests that lower 2D:4D ratio men do find their way into the Premier and 1st Divisions more frequently than players with relatively high ratios. Of course there is also competition within clubs to progress from the youth squads to a regular first team place. Many young players are not retained at age 18 years, while others go on to the reserves or to be regarded as a first-team player. The mean ratio of the left hand of the youth

Table 9.3. English Football League players honored at the 100th anniversary

Player	Clubs	Playing Career
Ossie Ardilles	Tottenham Hotspur, Blackburn Rovers, QPR, Swindon Town	1954 –1971
Jimmy Armfield	Blackpool	1954–1971
John Barnes	Watford, Liverpool, Newcastle United	1981–1998
John Charles	Swansea City, Leeds Utd, Cardiff City	1948–1966
Ray Clemence	Scunthorpe United, Liverpool, Tottenham Hotspur	1965–1988
Kenny Dalglish	Liverpool	1977–1990
Tom Finney	Preston North End	1946–1960
Trevor Francis	Birmingham City, Nottingham Forrest, Manchester City, QPR, Sheffield Wednesday	1970–1995
Paul Gascoigne	Newcastle United, Tottenham Hotspur, Middlesbrough	1984–1998
Johnny Giles	Manchester United, Leeds United, West Bromwich Albion	1959–1977
George Hardwick	Middlesbrough, Oldham Athletic	1937–1956
Johnny Haynes	Fulham	1952–1970
Glenn Hoddle	Tottenham Hotspur, Swindon Town, Chelsea	1974–1996
Norman Hunter	Leeds United, Bristol City, Barnsley	1962–1983
Geoff Hurst	West Ham United, Stoke City, West Bromwich Albion	1959–1976
Pat Jennings	Watford, Tottenham Hotspur, Arsenal	1962–1985
Cliff Jones	Swansea City, Tottenham Hotspur, Fulham	1952–1970
Nat Lofthouse	Bolton Wanderers	1946–1961
Dave Mackay	Tottenham Hotspur, Derby County, Swindon Town	1958–1972
Wilf Mannion	Middlesbrough, Hull City	1936–1956
Stanley Matthews	Stoke City, Blackpool	1931–1966
Paul McGrath	Manchester United, Aston Villa, Derby County	1981–1998
Frank McLintock	Leicester City, Arsenal, QPR	1959–1977
Alan Mullery	Fulham, Tottenham Hotspur	1958–1976
Terry Paine	Southampton, Hereford United	1956–1977
Bryan Robson	West Bromwich Albion, Manchester United, Middlesbrough	1978–1990
Joe Royle	Everton	1963–1978
Len Shackleton	Bradford Park Avenue, Newcastle United, Sunderland	1946–1958
Alan Shearer	Southampton, Blackburn Rovers, Newcastle United	1987–1998
Peter Shilton	Leicester City, Stockport County, Nottingham Forest, Southampton	1965–1997
Tommy Smith	Liverpool, Swansea City	1962–1979

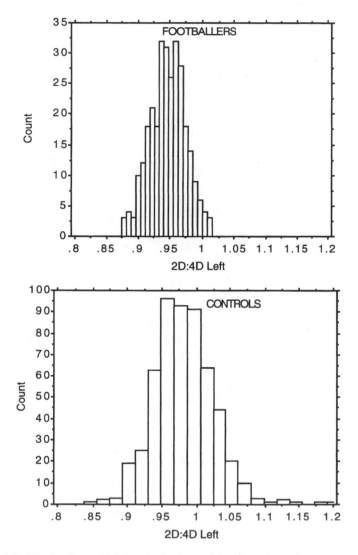

Figure 9.3. Distributions of left-hand 2D:4D in professional football players and male controls recruited from the Merseyside area. Most of the players (90%) had 2D:4D ratios of less than 0.98 which is the male mean in northwest England. The proportion in the controls of less than 0.98 was 50%. Therefore, the sample of players showed a higher percentage of male-type ratios than controls (left-hand players 0.95 ± 0.03, controls 0.98 ± 0.04, t = 13.12, p = 0.0001 Bonferroni adjusted p = 0.0001; right-hand players 0.95 ± 0.03, controls 0.98 ± 0.04, t = 12.24, p = 0.0001).

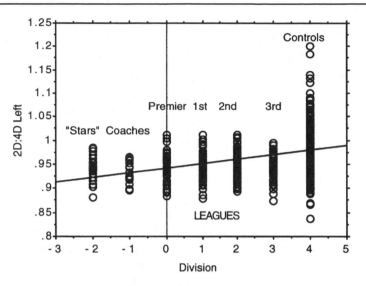

Figure 9.4. The 2D:4D ratios of the left hand progressively increase from "stars," i.e., a sample of elite international players, through professional coaches, to Premier League, 1st, 2nd, and 3rd Division players, to controls who do not play professional football ($b = 0.009$, $F = 163.02$, $p = 0.0001$). This suggests that professional football players of the very highest level of ability have experienced high levels of testosterone in utero.

squads was 0.95 ± 0.03 while the first-team players had lower mean ratios (0.94 ± 0.02) and the reserves higher ratios (0.96 ± 0.03, these differences were significant ANOVA, $F = 5.48$, $p = 0.005$). It appears that progression to a first-team place is associated with low 2D:4D ratios, but those players ranked as of "reserve" standard had higher ratios. It is likely that young players judged to be below professional standard will have higher ratios than their colleagues who progress further. A simultaneous regression analysis with dependent variable left 2D:4D and independent variables division and first team or reserves showed that first-team players had lower 2D:4D ratios than reserves independent of the division in which they were playing (first team $= 1$, reserves $= 2$, $b = 0.01$, $t = 2.69$, $p = 0.008$). The relationship between 2D:4D and division remained positive but was now nonsignificant ($b = 0.002$, $t = 1.48$, $p = 0.14$). This analysis indicates that progression to a secure first-team place is indeed related to low 2D:4D ratio and that competition within clubs is in a sense more frequent and intense than that afforded by transfer of players between clubs.

2D:4D in Players Who Had Represented Their Country

To play for one's country is one measure of high ability. International appearances are counted in "caps." Of course not all caps are equal in terms of indicating ability. Countries differ in their population base and in interest in football. Those nations, such as England, in which football is a very popular sport have intense competition for caps. The frequency of international matches also varies from country to country. This means that numbers of caps per player may not be an equal measure of ability between countries. In the sample we had 37 players who had reached the end of their career or were near the end, and had played for one of the home countries. There were also 227 players who, judging from their place of birth, would also qualify to represent either England, Scotland, Wales, Northern Ireland, or Eire. The left-hand 2D:4D ratio of the international group was significantly lower than that of the noninternationals (internationals 0.94 ± 0.02, noninternationals 0.95 ± 0.03, $t = 2.47$, $p = 0.01$). Left-hand 2D:4D ratio also showed a negative but nonsignificant association with log transformed number of international caps ($b = -5.55$, $F = 2.25$, $p = 0.07$ one-tailed). That is, there was an indication that players with low ratios had higher numbers of caps. The effect of country was controlled in a simultaneous regression analysis with log transformed number of caps as the dependent variable (country was dummy coded: England $= 1$, Scotland $= 2$, Wales $= 3$, Northern Ireland $= 4$, Eire $= 5$). Number of international caps was now weakly but significantly predicted by left-hand 2D:4D ratio ($b = -6.29$, $t = 1.72$, $p = 0.045$ one-tailed). It was not possible to predict a priori the direction of differences in 2D:4D ratio between players from different countries. One would be foolhardy and probably chauvinistic to attempt such an exercise. The positive relationship between country and international caps was not significant at the two-tailed level ($b = 0.14$, $t = 1.77$, $p = 0.08$). Comparative measures of 2D:4D between international squads of players would be of great interest and may prove to be predictive of success in international competitions such as the World Cup.

In the context of between-nations variation in football ability, it is instructive to compare the 2D:4D ratio of black players in the sample to their Caucasian colleagues. Black players were rare in the English league competitions up to the 1960s. They are much more common now, indicating welcome evidence of diminishing racial prejudice. Surprisingly our sample contained only 13 black players, i.e., less than 1% of the sample. This is probably because we sampled from clubs in areas with traditionally few black residents. Despite the low proportion of black participants in the sample, the difference in mean 2D:4D between black and Caucasian players was highly significant (black players 0.93 ± 0.02; Caucasian players 0.95 ± 0.03, $t = 3.28$, $p = 0.001$). There is little doubt that the English game is enriched by the presence of black players. Managers and scouts should be aware that low 2D:4D ratios may indicate potential for great football talent within this group.

2D:4D Ratio in Aspiring Football Players

We do not yet know whether 2D:4D ratio predicts a significant proportion of the variance of football ability within a sample of professional football players. Our problem in assessing the predictive power of 2D:4D is that football ability is a matter of opinion. However, the trend in figure 9.3 and other evidence suggests it may well do. If so, the 2D:4D ratio could be used to select young players who have not yet developed fully (2D:4D is fixed at birth). Identifying prepubertal players who are likely to be exceptional players after puberty is difficult. Competition for schoolboy international places is very strong. Despite this, few schoolboy internationals progress to places in the full international team. Early selection could facilitate coaching. I would stress that the ratio must be used as an addition to the judgment of coaches. Low 2D:4D is unlikely to be a strong indicator of football ability in a randomly selected group of males. However, in a sample of young males who have not yet entered puberty and who show some football ability, it may provide an additional discriminator that helps to predict ability. Other intriguing implications may arise if 2D:4D predicts football ability. There are known geographical differences in mean ratios. Some countries have higher proportions of low 2D:4D males than others. Given similar population levels, the former countries may find it easier to select high-ability football players than the latter.

Conclusions

The studies considered in this chapter suggest that low 2D:4D is (a) associated with success in a range of sports; (b) related to good visual-spatial perception; (c) a characteristic of professional football players; (d) found in first-team football players compared to reserves; and (e) a characteristic of international players compared to noninternationals.

What has been done for a sport such as football can be done for other sports and for athletic disciplines. Within groups of sportsmen and athletes 2D:4D ratios may be strong predictors of pace, endurance, and visual-spatial abilities. It remains to be seen how far this can take us in the identification and encouragement of young talented sports people and athletes.

CHAPTER 10

2nd to 4th Digit Ratio
and Future Research

I have tried to give a picture of present research into 2D:4D ratio. Where should we go from here? Clearly there is much to do. In this chapter I select and emphasize some of the lines of inquiry which may be fruitful in future research into the ratio.

Sex, Ethnicity, Species, and Higher Taxa Differences in 2D:4D

I think it is now well established that 2D:4D ratio is sexually dimorphic in its expression. It is more of a surprise that the ratio also shows geographical and ethnic differences in human populations. These need to be defined and related, where possible, to environmental and cultural variables. What is the pattern of 2D:4D ratio among Orientals, Australian Aboriginals, Asians, and North, Central, and South American indigenous peoples? What is the detail of the 2D:4D patterns among Europeans and among African groups? Can we relate 2D:4D ratio to diets rich in fat? Are there extreme ratios in northern populations where lipid intake is high? Are there subtle changes across short distances within countries? For example, Italy is a nation that has a long linear shape. Are there clinal differences in 2D:4D ratio in a north-south transect of Italy? These are questions of theoretical and practical importance, for they bear on considerations of absolute concentrations of prenatal testosterone and estrogen.

Related to questions of population differences are evolutionary relationships between the 2D:4D ratios of our close ancestors the primates (particularly the apes) and patterns of human 2D:4D ratio. Does 2D:4D vary between arboreal and terrestrial groups? Does the taxonomic pattern of 2D:4D ratio shed light on how early human populations differentiated and where they differentiated? These questions then lead to sexual dimorphism in 2D:4D ratio in mammals and tetrapods in general. Is there evidence for an ancient relationship between 2D:4D, sexual dimorphism, *Hox* genes for limb and gonad development, and the origin of the pentadactyl limb?

Prenatal Conditions and 2D:4D

What of the question of the 2D:4D ratio and prenatal hormone levels? This is fundamental to our interpretations of what the 2D:4D ratio is about.

Prenatal conditions are difficult to monitor, but we should make efforts to confirm the link between low 2D:4D and in utero testosterone and high 2D:4D ratio and prenatal estrogen. In this way we can make sense of the major population differences in 2D:4D ratio. Is it really the case that Jamaican, Finnish, and Zulu men are exposed to much more testosterone in utero than English, Spanish, and Polish men? Are English, Spanish, and Polish women exposed to much more prenatal estrogen than Jamaican, Finnish, and Zulu women? What of the differences between the sexes of different groups? Why is the 2D:4D ratio of English males higher than the ratio of Jamaican females? The differences may not arise from absolute concentrations of prenatal hormones. Rather they may spring from population differences in the distribution and frequency of androgen and estrogen receptors. Between-group differences in 2D:4D ratio point to very strong selection pressures. Perhaps a combination of local dietary preferences, immune challenges, and mating systems can explain at least some of this fascinating geographical and ethnic variation.

2D:4D and Status

The 2D:4D ratio may illuminate the difficult areas of assertiveness and aggression. I think the data suggesting relationships between the ratio and these types of behaviors are at present weak. This may stem from the fact that testosterone and estrogen themselves have only weak effects on these traits. We must proceed with caution here. The possibility that 2D:4D is negatively correlated with deprivation scores is fascinating, but it needs confirmation across a number of cultures. Of course, concepts such as socioeconomic status may be related to complex social factors and may not be determined primarily or even weakly by biological variables. However, it is tempting to say that high male testosterone, low 2D:4D ratios, and high fertility are related to low socioeconomic status and high deprivation. In support of this, high testosterone has been correlated with low occupational achievement (Dabbs 1992). My feeling is that 2D:4D ratio will provide valuable data in these areas, but much further work is needed.

2D:4D and Fertility

Are 2D:4D ratios related to lifetime reproductive success? I think the data presented in chapter 4 indicates a weak but nevertheless real relationship. Correlates of fertility traits such as sperm counts and hormone concentrations are not necessarily going to be associated with lifetime reproductive success. Many influences may intervene and obscure such an association, for example, the fertility of one's partner, the availability of effective birth control, and the preferred number of children. If male 2D:4D is negatively related to lifetime reproductive success and female 2D:4D positively related to lifetime reproductive success, these opposing effects may limit directional selection toward low or high 2D:4D ratio. We need more data from more populations. At present our data suggest that the negative relationship of male 2D:4D and reproductive success is robust, but perhaps the female positive association does not extend to populations that have a low mean 2D:4D ratio. If so, it means that a potentially important stabilizing influence on selection for lower 2D:4D ratio will be ineffective. This highlights the questions regarding why populations have different mean 2D:4D ratios and what theoretical framework we need to understand between-population variation. I have chosen to use the concept of sexually antagonistic genes in an attempt to model the evolution of these between-population differences. It may be that this approach is essentially correct, in which case there will be repeated cycles of invasion of genes coding for low 2D:4D phenotypes followed by the spread of genes for high 2D:4D phenotypes. Alternatively, there may be a few environmental and mating system variables that result in directional selection to either extreme of the 2D:4D spectrum or in stabilizing selection. It is important we get the theoretical framework right. For this we need more empirical work in order that our theoretical models are well founded and adequately tested.

2D:4D and the Central Nervous System

What of the deleterious effects of prenatal testosterone on the developing brain? Low 2D:4D, particularly low ratios in males, may be related to a reduction in verbal fluency, an increased probability of autism, and a tendency toward depression. These conclusions need to be confirmed and extended to other deleterious traits such as dyslexia, migraine, and stammering (Geschwind and Galaburda 1985a, 1985b, 1985c). A likely correlate of 2D:4D ratio is schizophrenia. The prognosis for this illness is worse for men compared to women. It may be that age at presentation, severity of symptoms, and perhaps type of symptom such as the hearing of voices may be predicted by 2D:4D ratio. I expect that schizophrenics will have low 2D:4D ratios compared to population norms.

It is unlikely that 2D:4D is related to IQ. Much of what is sexually dimorphic has been eliminated from IQ scores. However, the relationship between 2D:4D and different types of academic ability may be strong. Mathematicians, physicists, and engineers are likely to have low 2D:4D compared to historians and language graduates. Within disciplines such as mathematics and physics 2D:4D is likely to be negatively associated with final degree classification. Within the arts and humanities, 2D:4D may be a positive predictor of examination success.

2D:4D and Major Diseases

The 2D:4D ratio may prove to be a valuable predictor of high-risk individuals for major diseases such as breast cancer, ovarian cancer, myocardial infarction, type II diabetes, prostate cancer, lung and colon cancer, malaria, tuberculosis, and susceptibility to infection by HIV and progression to AIDS. Associated with this is the necessity to examine the relationship between 2D:4D and immunocompetence. This may be done by correlating the expression of 2D:4D with such things as the concentration of the major immunoglobulin classes IgG, IgM, and IgA, the function of histocompatibility antigens (which complex with and present antigens on the surface of lymphocytes), the levels of complement (a complex of proteins that produce an enzymatic amplifying cascade which leads to the lysis of bacteria), the concentrations of types of complement (e.g., the complement fragments C3a, C4a, and C5a cause the release of inflammatory mediators from mast cells and C5b, C6, C7, C8, and C9 are involved in the reaction that perforates cell membranes), and the percentage of monocytes (a type of macrophage in the blood which is able to engulf microorganisms; Gell et al. 1974, and for a review of immune system function, see Delves and Roitt 2000). Alternatively, relationships between 2D:4D and such diseases as onchocerciasis and malaria can be investigated. Small-scale clinal changes in the values of 2D:4D within ethnic groups may be related to the historical frequency of parasitic diseases in, say, wet lowland and well-drained upland areas. In this respect the frequency of traits such as sickle cell anemia, a mutation that is at high frequency in malarial areas, may be correlated with variation in 2D:4D.

There are already preliminary data for the relationship between 2D:4D and myocardial infarction and breast cancer. More work is urgently needed on 2D:4D and the etiology of these diseases. Lifestyle interventions and early detection may be facilitated by large-scale programs of 2D:4D measurement. In this work it is essential that we establish a "worldwide atlas" of 2D:4D patterns. Patterns of disease may show very considerable geographical heterogeneity. Such geographical variation is often not predicted by known risk factors that affect disease expression within groups. Knowledge of between-group differences in 2D:4D expression may enable us to explain some of the geographical heterogeneity in major diseases.

The 2D:4D ratio may shed some light on the fetal origins of adult-onset disease. The innovative work of Barker (1992) and his colleagues has established links between low birth weight and many adult-onset traits, including coronary artery disease mortality and morbidity, insulin resistance, impaired glucose tolerance, type II diabetes, blood pressure, plasma fibrinogen, and factor VII levels (for a review of this field, see Jarvelin 2000). Low 2D:4D may be associated with lower than expected birth weight but also a reduced risk of premature myocardial infarction in men. These relationships seem to be in conflict with one another. Further work on 2D:4D and measures of fetal growth is essential. It may be that prenatal steroid levels can be more influential than normal variation in maternal diet in the control of fetal growth.

2D:4D and Sexual Orientation

What of the contentious issue of sexual orientation? Is the prenatal ratio of testosterone to estrogen important in establishing human sexual orientation? This is a question that work on 2D:4D ratio may help answer. It is important to confirm whether female and male gays have different 2D:4D ratios than heterosexual women and men. Childhood gender nonconformity is a predictor of homosexuality. It would be of great interest to establish whether 2D:4D predicts gender-specific behavior in children. In this work we must be careful to control for ethnic variation. We must also be sensitive to the implications of theories of hormonal determination of sexual orientation. Female and male homosexuality may be precipitated by high concentrations of prenatal testosterone. However, it is important to establish whether testosterone levels have to be (a) higher than expected for that particular geographical/ethnic group or (b) above a certain absolute level. If it is (b) then the frequency of homosexuality will vary from group to group.

2D:4D, Male Displays, and Male:Male Competition

The 2D:4D ratios may also tell us much about what information is present in human male displays and male:male competition. I think that women may be sensitive to any evidence of high in utero testosterone concentrations in men. Displays of musical ability and visual-spatial ability are likely to be very attractive to women because they are difficult to fake and because they correlate with male fertility. Orchestras and bands may share real affinities with leks in nonhuman species. That is, they are groups of displaying males that attract large numbers of females. In this context what of religion and 2D:4D ratio? Is this a step too far? It is a popular conception that charismatic religious figures are often male and often have many sexual partners. Darwin (1871) included impassioned oratory with music in his list of sexually appealing traits. Leaders of sects and other charismatic religious figures may have low 2D:4D ratios.

Male-oriented human sport may also be merely demonstrations of high fertility and resource-holding potential. Good visual-spatial ability and vascular systems are necessary for success in most sports. Boxing, fencing, soccer, American football, baseball, and motor racing test one or both of these traits. It will be instructive to explore whether 2D:4D ratios of young men may help predict their eventual level of success in their favorite sports.

I suppose one reaction to this program for research is to say that a trivial trait such as 2D:4D ratio is not going to be predictive in such a wide-ranging agenda. My answer is that 2D:4D is a marker for the prenatal conditions associated with the establishment of sex differences. Sex differences reach into every aspect of our lives. From our fertility, to the kinds of diseases we are prone to, and to the behaviors that we show, sexual dimorphism is often apparent but often ignored. I hope my arguments have some truth to them. In this I am content to wait and see where the data lead us.

Bibliography

Adams, M. R., J. K. Williams, and J. R. Kaplan. 1995. Effects of androgens on coronary atherosclerosis and athersclerosis-related impairment of vascular responsiveness. *Arteriosclerosis Thrombosis Vascular Biology* 15:562–570.

Ainbender, E., R. Weisinger, M. Hevizy, and H. L. Hodes. 1968. Differences in immunoglobulin class of polio antibody in the serum of men and women. *Journal of Immunology* 101:92–98.

Aksut, S. V., G. Aksut, A. Karamehmetoglu, and E. Oram. 1986. The determination of serum estradiol, testosterone, and progesterone in acute myocardial infarction. *Japanese Heart Journal* 27:825–837.

Alexandersen, P., J. Haarbo, I. Byrialsen, H. Lawaetz, and C. Christiansen. 1999. Natural androgens inhibit male atherosclerosis: A study in castrated, cholesterolfed rabbits. *Circulation Research* 84:813–819.

American Psychiatric Association. 1994. *Diagnostic and Statistical Manual of Mental Disorders.* 4th ed. Washington, D.C.: APA.

Anderson, T. J., S. Battersby, R.J.B. King, K. McPherson, and J. J. Going. 1989. Oral contraceptive use influences resting breast proliferation. *Human Pathology* 20:1139–1144.

Archer, J. 1991. The influence of testosterone on human aggression. *British Journal of Psychology* 82:1–28.

Archer, J. 1994. Testosterone and aggression. *Journal of Offender Rehabilitation* 21:3–25.

Archer, J., J. Kilpatrick, and R. Bramwell. 1995. Comparison of two aggression inventories. *Aggressive Behavior* 21:371–380.

Arrieta, I., B. Martinez, B. Criado, and B. Lobato. 1993. Ridge hypoplasia and ridge dissociation: Minor physical anomalies in autistic children. *Clinical Genetics* 44:107–108.

Bailey, M. J., and R. C. Pillard. 1991. A genetic study of male sexual orientation. *Archives of General Psychiatry* 12:1089–1096.

Bailey, M. J., and J. J. Zucker. 1995. Childhood sex-typed behavior and sexual orientation: A conceptual analysis and quantitative review. *Developmental Psychology* 31:43–55.

Bailey, P. 2000. The generation gap: Twenty years of HIV and AIDS. *Wellcome News* 23:14–15.

Bailey. T., A. Le Couteur, I. Gottesman, P. Bolton, E. Simonoff, E. Yuzda, and M. Rutter. 1995. Autism as a strongly genetic disorder: Evidence from a British twin study. *Psychological Medicine* 25:63–77.

Baker, F. 1888. Anthropological notes on the human hand. *American Anthropologist* 1:51–76.

Banks, T., and J. M. Dabbs. 1996. Salivary testosterone and cortisol in a delinquent and violent urban subculture. *Journal of Social Psychology* 136:49–56.

Bardin, C. W., and C. F. Caterall. 1981. Testosterone: A major determinant of extragenital sexual dimorphism. *Science* 211:1285–1294.

Barker, D.J.B. 1986. Infant mortality, childhood nutrition, and ischaemic heart disease in England and Wales. *Lancet* 1:1077–1081.

Barker, D.J.B. 1995. Fetal origins of coronary heart disease. *British Medical Journal* 311:171–174.

Barker, D.J.B. (Ed.). 1992. *Fetal and Infant Origins of Adult Disease*. London: British Medical Journal Publishing Group.

Barker, D.J.B., and C. Osmond. 1986. Infant mortality, childhood nutrition, and ischaemic heart disease in England and Wales. *Lancet* (i) 1077–1081.

Baron-Cohen, S. 1995. *Mindblindness: An Essay on Autism and Theory of Mind*. Cambridge, Mass.: MIT Press/Bradford Books.

Baron-Cohen, S., and P. Bolton. 1993. *Autism: The Facts*. Oxford: Oxford University Press.

Baron-Cohen, S., and J. Hammer. 1997. Is autism an extreme form of the male brain? *Advances in Infancy Research* 11:193–217.

Baron-Cohen, S., S. Wheelwright, C. Stott, P. Bolton, and I. Goodyer. 1997. Is there a link between engineering and autism? *Autism* 1:101–109.

Barnard, C. J., J. M. Behnke, and A. R. Gage. 1998. The role of parasite-induced immunodepression, rank, and social environment in the modulation of behaviour and hormone concentration in male laboratory mice (*Mus musculus*). *Proceedings of the Royal Society of London, B Series*, 693–701.

Barrett-Connor, E. 1995. Testosterone and risk factors for cardiovascular disease in men. *Diabetes Metabolism* 21:156–161.

Barrett-Connor, E., and K. S. Kaw. 1988. Endogenous sex hormone levels and cardiovascular disease in men: A prospective population-based study. *Circulation* 78:539–543.

Barrett-Connor, E., T. Khaw, and S.C.C. Yen. 1986. A prospective study of dehydroepiandrostenone sulphate, mortality and cardio-vascular disease. *New England Journal of Medicine* 315:1519–1524.

Beck, A. T., and R. A. Steer. 1984. Internal consistencies of the original and revised Beck Depression Inventory. *Journal of Clinical Psychology* 40:1365–1367.

Bell, A. P., M. S. Weinberg, and S. K. Hammersmith. 1981. *Sexual Preference: Its Development in Men and Women*. Bloomington: Indiana University Press.

Bell, G. H., D. Emslie-Smith, and C. R. Paterson. 1980. *BDS Textbook of Physiology*. 10th ed. Edinburgh: Churchill Livingstone.

Bettelheim, B. 1967. *The Empty Fortress: Infantile Autism and the Birth of the Self*. New York: Free Press.

Bjorntorp, P. 1991. Adipose tissue distribution and functions. *International Journal of Obesity* 15:67–87.

Blanchard, R. 1997. Birth order and sibling sex ratio in homosexual and heterosexual males and females. *Annual Review of Sex Research* 8:27–67.

Blanchard, R., and A. F. Bogaert. 1996. Homosexuality in men and number of older brothers. *American Journal of Psychiatry* 153:27–31, 1996.

Bogaert, A. F., and S. Hershberger. 1999. The relation between sexual orientation and penile size. *Archives of Sexual Behavior* 28:213–221.

Bolton, P., H. MacDonald, A. Pickles, P. Rios, S. Goode, M. Crowson, A. Bailey, and M. Rutter. 1994. A case-control family history study of autism. *Journal of Child Psychology and Psychiatry* 35:877–900.

Boyd Eaton, S., M. C. Pike, R. V. Short, N. C. Lee, R. A. Hatcher, J. W. Wood, C. M. Wothman, N. G. Blurton Jones, M. J. Konner, K. R. Hill, R. Bailey, and A. M. Hurtado. 1994. Women's reproductive cancers in evolutionary context. *Quarterly Review of Biology* 69:353–365.

Brabin, B. J. 1991. An assessment of low birth-weight risk in primiparae as an indicator of malaria control in pregnancy. *International Journal of Epidemiology* 20:276–283.

Brabin, L. 1990. Sex differentials in susceptibility to lymphatic filariasis and implications for maternal-child immunity. *Epidemiology and Infection* 105:335–353.

Brabin, L., and B. J. Brabin. 1992. Parasitic infections in women and their consequences. *Advances in Parasitology* 31:1–81.

Brandling-Bennett, A. D., J. Anderson, H. Fuglsang, and R. Collins. 1981. Onchocerciasis in Guatemala: Epidemiology in fincas with various intensities of infection. *American Journal of Tropical Medicine and Hygeine* 30:970–981.

Brinton, L. A., C. Schairer, R. N. Hoover, and J. F. Fraumeni. 1988. Menstrual factors and risk of breast cancer. *Cancer Investigations* 6:245–254.

British Heart Foundation. 1996. *British Heart Foundation Statistics Database*, 21–22.

Brodie, H.K.H., N. Gartrell, C. Doering, and T. Rhue. 1974. Plasma testosterone levels in heterosexual and homosexual men. *American Journal of Psychiatry* 131:82–83.

Brown, P.J.B., and P.W.J. Batey. 1987. A national classification of 1981 Census Enumeration Districts: A derivation of Super Profile Area Types. *Area Classification Note 1*. Liverpool, England: Liverpool University.

Bryden, M. P., I. C. McManus, and M. B. Bulman-Fleming. 1994. Evaluating the empirical support for the Geschwind-Behan-Galaburda model of cerebral lateralisation. *Brain and Cognition* 26:103–167.

Buck, G. M., D. L. Cookfair, and A. M. Michalek. 1989. Intrauterine growth retardation and risk of sudden infant death syndrome. *American Journal of Epidemiology* 129:874–884.

Burkitt, D., and G. T. O'Connor. 1961. Malignant lymphoma in African children. *Cancer* 14:258–269.

Burns, E. M., K. H. Arehart, and S. L. Campbell. 1992. Prevalence of spontaneous otoacoustic emissions in neonates. *Journal of the Acoustical Society of America* 91:1571–1575.

Burns, E. M., S. L. Campbell, and K. H. Arehart. 1994. Longitudinal measurements of spontaneous otoacoustic emissions in infants. *Journal of the Acoustical Society of America* 95:385–394.

Burt, A. 1995. Perspective: The evolution of fitness. *Evolution* 49:1–8.

Buss, D. M. 1985. Human mate selection. *American Scientist* 73:47–51.

Butterworth, M. B., B. McClellan, and M. Alansmith. 1967. Influence of sex on immunoglobulin levels. *Nature* 214:1224–1225.

Campbell, M., B. Geller, A. M. Small, T. A. Petti, and S. H. Ferris. 1978. Minor physical anomalies in young psychotic children. *American Journal of Psychiatry* 135:573–575.

Campbell, S. 1989. The detection of intrauterine growth retardation. In *RCOG Study Groups Proceedings: Fetal Growth,* ed. F. Sharp, R. B. Fraser, and R. D. Milner. London: Royal College of Obstetricians and Gynaecologists.

Casanova, G. 1997. *The History of My Life.* Trans. W. R. Trask. Baltimore: Johns Hopkins University Press.

Cengiz, K., M. Alvur, and U. Dindar. 1991. Serum creatine phosphokinase, lactic dehydrogenase, estradiol, progesterone and testosterone levels in male patients with acute myocardial infarction and unstable angina pectoris. *Materia Medica Polona* 23:195–198.

Chandler, C. R. 1995. Practical considerations in the use of simultaneous inference for multiple tests. *Animal Behaviour* 49:524–527.

Coates, M. 1996. The Devonian tetrapod *Acanthostega gunnari Jarvik*: Postcranial anatomy, basal tetrapod interrelationships and patterns of skeletal evolution. *Transactions Royal Society of Edinburgh-Earth Sciences* 87:363–372.

Cohen, J. A. 1992. A power primer. *Psychology Bulletin* 112:155–159.

Coleman, M., and J. P. Blass. 1985. Autism and lactic acidosis. *Journal of Autism and Developmental Disorders* 15:1–8.

Dabbs, J. M., Jr. 1992. Testosterone and occupational achievement. *Social Forces* 70:813–824.

Dabbs, J. M., G. L. Jurkovic, and R. L. Frady. 1995. Saliva testosterone and cortisol among late adolescent juvenile offenders. *Journal of Abnormal Child Psychology* 19:469–478.

Daly, M., and M. Wilson. 1994. Evolutionary psychology of male violence. In *Male Violence*, ed. J. Archer. London: Routledge, 253–288.

Danforth, C. H. 1921. Distribution of hair on the digits in man. *American Journal of Physical Anthropology* 4:189–204.

Darwin, C. 1871. *The Descent of Man, and Selection in Relation to Sex.* London: Raven Press.

David, D., and R. Brannon. 1976. The male sex role: Our culture's blueprint for manhood and what it's done for us lately. In *The Forty-nine Percent Majority: The Male Sex Role,* ed. D. David and R. Brannon. Reading, Mass.: Addison Wesley.

Davies, R. H., B. Harris, D. R. Thomas, N. Cook, G. Read, and D. Riad-Fahmy. 1992. Salivary testosterone levels and major depressive illness in men. *British Journal of Psychiatry* 161:629–632.

Delves, P. J., and I. M. Roitt. 2000. The immune system. *New England Journal of Medicine* 343:37–49.

Dickey, R. P., and R. F. Gasser. 1993. Ultrasound evidence for variability in the size and development of normal human embryos before the tenth post-insemination week after assisted reproductive technologies. *Human Reproduction* 8:331–337.

Doerr, P., K. M. Pirke, G. Kockott, and F. Dittmar. 1976. Further studies on sex hormones in male homosexuals. *Archives of General Psychiatry* 33:611–614.

Dorner, G., F. Rohde, F. Stahl, L. Krell, and W. Masius. 1975. A neuroendocrine predisposition for homosexuality in men. *Archives of Sexual Behaviour* 4:1–8.

Ecker, A. 1875. Einige bemekungen uber einen schwankengen charakter in der hand des menschen. *Archives fur Anthropologie (Braunschweig)* 8:67–75.

Elledge, R. M., and C. K. Osborne. 1997. Oestrogen receptors and breast cancer. *British Medical Journal* 314:1843–1844.

Ellis, L., and H. Nyborg. 1992. Racial/ethnic variations in male testosterone levels: A probable contributor to group differences in health. *Steroids* 57:72–75.

English, K. M., O. Mandour, R. P. Steeds, M. J. Diver, T. H. Jones, and K. S. Channer. 2000. Men with coronary artery disease have lower levels of androgens than men with normal coronary angiograms. *European Heart Journal* 21:890–894.

Entrican, J. H., C. Beach, D. D. Carroll, A. Klopper, M. Mackie, M., and A. S. Douglas. 1978. Raised plasma oestradiol and oestrone levels in young survivors of myocardial infarction. *Lancet* 2:487–490.

Evans, D. J., R. G. Hoffmann, R. K. Kalkhoff, and A. H. Kissebah. 1982. Body fat topography and skeletal muscle insulin resistance in obese women. *Diabetes* 31:161–164.

Evans, D. J., R. G. Hoffmann, R. K. Kalkhoff, and A. H. Kissebah. 1983. Relation-ship of androgenic activity to body fat topography, fat cell morphology and meta-bolic aberrations in premenstrual women. *Journal of Clinical Endocrinology and Metabolism* 57:304–310.

Evers, S., J. Dannert, D. Rodding, G. Rotter, and E. Bernd-Ringelstein. 1999. The cerebral haemodynamics of music perception: A transcranial Doppler sonography study. *Brain* 122:75–85.

Fchifter, T. 1994. Neuroimaging in infantile autism. *Journal of Child Neurology* 92:155–161.

Finegan, J. K., B. Bartelman, and P. Y. Wong. 1991. A window for the study of pre-natal sex influences on postnatal development. *Journal of Genetic Psychology* 150:101–112.

Fisher, R. A. 1930. *The Genetical Theory of Natural Selection.* London: Clarendon Press.

Friedman, R. C., I. Dyrenfurth, D. Linkie, R. Tendler, and J. L. Fliess. 1977. Hor-mones and sexual orientation in men. *American Journal of Psychiatry* 134:571–572.

Frith, U. 1989. *Autism: Explaining the Enigma.* Oxford: Basil Blackwell.

Gacono, C. 2000. *The Clinical and Forensic Assessment of Psychopathy: A Practitioner's Guide.* Mahwah, N.J.: Lawrence Erlbaum.

Gangestad, S. W., and R. Thornhill. 1997. Human sexual selection and development stability. In J. A. Simpson and D. T. Kenrick (eds.), *Evolutionary Personality and Social Psychology,* 169–195. Hillsdale NJ: Erlbaum.

Garn, S. M. 1951. The use of middle phalangeal hair in population studies. *American Journal of Physical Anthropology* 9:325–333.

Garn, S. M. 1957. Fat weight and fat placement in the female. *Science* 125:1091–1093.

Garn, S. M., A. R. Burdi, W. J. Babler, and S. Stinson. 1975. Early prenatal attain-ment of adult metacarpal-phalangeal rankings and proportions. *American Journal of Physical Anthropolology* 43:327–332.

Gateley, C. A. 1998. Male breast disease. *The Breast* 7:121–127.

Gell, P.G.H., R.R.A. Coombs, and P. J. Lachmann. 1974. *Clinical Aspects of Immunol-ogy.* 3d ed. Oxford: Blackwell.

George, F. W., J. E. Griffin, M. Leshin, and J. D. Wilson. 1981. Endocrine control of sexual differentiation in the human. In *Fetal Endocrinology,* ed. M. J Novy and J. A. Resko. New York: Academic Press, 341–357.

George, R. 1930. Human finger types. *Anatomical Record* 46:199–204.

Geschwind, N., and A. M. Galaburda. 1985a. Cerebral lateralisation. Biological mechanisms, associations and pathology: I. A hypothesis and a program for research. *Archives of Neurology* 42:428–459.

Geschwind, N., and A. M. Galaburda. 1985b. Cerebral lateralisation. Biological mechanisms, associations and pathology: II. A hypothesis and a program for research. *Archives of Neurology* 42:521–552.

Geschwind, N., and A. M. Galaburda. 1985c. Cerebral lateralisation. Biological mechanisms, associations and pathology: III. A hypothesis and a program for research. *Archives of Neurology* 42:634–654.

Geschwind, N., and A. M. Galaburda. 1987. *Cerebral Lateralization*. Cambridge, Mass.: MIT Press.

Gil, D., J. Graves, N. Hazon, and A. Wells. 1999. Male attractiveness and differential testosterone investment in zebra finch eggs. *Science* 286:126–128.

Gilger, J. W., B. F. Pennington, P. Green, S. A. Smith, and S. M. Smith. 1992. Dyslexia, immune disorders and left-handedness: Twin and family studies of their relations. *Neuropsychologia* 30:209–227.

Gilger, J. W., B. F. Pennington, R. J. Harbeck, J. C. DeFries, B. Kotzin, P. Green, and S. A. Smith. 1992. Twin and family study of the association between immune system dysfunction and dyslexia using blood serum immunoassay and survey data. *Brain and Cognition* 36:310–333.

Gilks, C. F. 1999. The challenge of HIV/AIDS in Sub-Saharan Africa. *Journal of Royal College of Physicians of London* 33:180–184.

Gladue, B. A. 1991. Aggressive behavioral characteristics, hormones, and sexual orientation in men and women. *Aggressive Behavior* 17:313–326.

Gladue, B. A., R. Green, and R. E. Hellman. 1984. Neuroendocrine response to estrogen and sexual orientation. *Science* 225:1496–1499.

Goedert, J. J., and W. A. Blattner. 1985. The epidemiology of AIDS and related conditions. In *AIDS: Etiology, Diagnosis and Prevention*, ed. V. T. Devita, S. Hellman, and S. A. Rosenberg. Philadelphia: Lippincott, 1–30.

Gooren, L. 1986. The neuroendocrine response of luteinising hormone to estrogen administration in heterosexual, homosexual and transsexual subjects. *Journal of Clinical Endocrinology and Metabolism* 63:583–588.

Gorman, M. R. 1984. Male homosexual desire: Neurological investigations and scientific bias. *Perspectives on Biology and Medicine* 38:61–81.

Grammer, K., and R. Thornhill. 1994. Human (*Homo sapiens*) facial attractiveness and sexual selection: The role of symmetry and averageness. *Journal of Comparative Psychology* 108:233–242.

Gray, H. 1858. *Anatomy: Descriptive and Surgical*. Bristol: Parragon.

Grimwood, A. 2000. We can do better than this: South Africa and AIDS drugs. *New Scientist* 166:44–45.

Gross-Isseroff, R., K. A. Dillon, M. Israeli, and A. Biegon. 1990. Regionally selective increases in mu opiod receptor density in the brains of suicide victims. *Brain Research* 530:312–316.

Grossman, C. 1989. Possible underlying mechanisms of sexual dimorphism in the immune response, fact and hypothesis. *Journal of Steroid Biochemistry* 34:241–251.

Gruning, J. 1886. Uber die lange der finger und zehen bei einigen volkerstammen. *Archives fur Anthropologie (Braunschweig)* 16:511–517.

Gualtieri, C. T., A. Adams, C. D. Shen, and D. Loiselle. 1982. Minor physical anomalies in alcoholic and schizophrenic adults and hyperactive and autistic children. *American Journal of Psychiatry* 139:640–643.

Haffner, S. M. 1996. Sex hormone binding protein, hyperinsulinaemia, insulin resistance and non-insulin-dependent diabetes. *Hormone Research* 45:233–237.

Haffner, S. M., R. D'Agostino, L. Mykkanen, R. Tracy, B. Howard, M. Rewers, J. Selby, P. J. Savage, and M. F. Saad. 1999. Insulin sensitivity in subjects with type II diabetes. Relationship to cardiovascular risk factors: The Insulin Resistance Atherosclerosis Study. *Diabetes Care* 22:562–568.

Haffner, S. M., L. Mykkanen, R. A. Valdez, and M. S. Katz. 1993. Relationship of sex hormones to lipids and lipoproteins in non-diabetic men. *Journal Clinical Endocrinology and Metabolism* 77:1610–1615.

Hall, J. A., and D. Kimura. 1994. Dermatoglyphic asymmetry and sexual orientation in men. *Behavioral Neuroscience* 8:1203–1206.

Halpern, D. F. 1992. *Sex Differences in Cognitive Abilities*. London: Lawrence Erlbaum Associates.

Hamalainen, E., H. Adlercreutz, C. Ehnholm, and P. Puska. 1986. Relationships of serum lipoproteins and apoproteins to sex hormones and to the binding capacity of sex hormone binding globulin in healthy Finnish men. *Metabolism* 35:535–541.

Hamer, D. H., and P. Copeland. 1994. *The Science of Desire*. New York: Simon and Schuster.

Hamer, D. H., S. Hu, V. L. Magnuson, N. Hu, and A.M.L. Pattatucci. 1993. A linkage between DNA markers on the X chromosome and male sexual orientation. *Science* 261:321–327.

Harris, M. 1989. *Our Kind*. New York: Harper and Row.

Heinonen, O. P., D. Slone, R. R. Monson, E. B. Hook, and S. Shapiro. 1977. Cardiovascular birth defects and antenatalexposure to female hormones. *New England Journal of Medicine* 296:67–70.

Hendricks, S. E., B. Graber, and J. F. Rodriguez-Sierra. 1989. Neuroendocrine responses to exogenous estrogen: No differences between heterosexual and homosexual men. *Psychoneuroendocrinology* 14:177–185.

Hepper, P. G., E. A. Shannon, and J. C. Dornan. 1997. Sex differences in fetal mouth movements. *Lancet* 350:1820.

Herault, Y., N. Fradeau, J. Zakany, and D. Duboule. 1997. *Ulnaless (Ul)*, a regulatory mutation inducing both loss-of-function and gain-of-function of posterior *Hoxd* genes. *Development* 124:3493–3500.

Heston, L. L., and J. Shields. 1968. Homosexuality in twins: A family study and registry study. *Archives of General Psychiatry* 18:149–160.

Hodgkin, J. 1991. Sex determination and the generation of sexually dimorphic nervous systems. *Neuron* 6:177–185.

Holden, C. 1986. Youth suicide: New research focuses on a growing social problem. *Science* 233:839–841.

Holst, K., E. Andersen, J. Phillip, and I. Henningsen. 1989. Antenatal and perinatal conditions correlated to handicap among four-year-old children. *American Journal of Perinatology* 6:258–267.

Holt, S. B. 1968. *The Genetics of Dermal Ridges.* Springfield, Ill.: Charles C. Thomas.

Hooper, E. 2000. *The River.* London: Allen Lane/Penguin Press.

Houle, D. 1992. Comparing evolvability and variability of traits. *Genetics* 130:195–204.

Hu, S., A.M.L. Pattatucci, C. Patterson, L. Li, D. W. Fulker, S. S. Cherny, L. Kruglyak, and D. H. Hamer. 1995. Linkage between sexual orientation and chromosome Xq28 in males but not in females. *Nature Genetics* 11:248–256.

Hume, D. K., and R. Montgomerie. 2001. Facial attractiveness signals different aspects of "quality" in women and men. *Evolution and Human Behavior* 22:92–112.

Hutchinson, G. E. 1959. A speculative consideration of certain possible forms of sexual selection in man. *American Naturalist* 93:81–91.

Hutchison, J. B., C. Beyer, R. E. Hutchison, and A. Wozniak. 1997. Sex differences in the regulation of embryonic aromatase. *Journal of Steroid Biochemistry and Molecular Biology* 61:315–322.

Hutton, J. L., P.O.D. Pharaoh, R.W.I. Cooke, and R. C. Stevenson. 1997. Differential effects of preterm birth and small gestational age on cognitive and motor development. *Archives of Disease in Childhood* 76:75–81.

Imagawa, W., J. Yang, R. Guzman, and S. Nandi. 1994. Control of mammary gland growth and differentiation. In *The Physiology of Reproduction*, vol. 2, ed. E. Knobil, J. D. Neill, G. S. Greenwald, C. L. Markert, and D. W. Pfaff. New York: Raven Press, 1033–1064.

Jamison, C. S., R. J. Meier, and B. C. Campbell. 1993. Dermatoglyphic asymmetry and testosterone levels in normal males. *American Journal of Physical Anthropology* 90:185–198.

Jarvelin, M. R. 2000. Congenital heart disease: Fetal and infant markers of adult heart disease. *Heart* 84:219–226.

Kallman, F. J. 1952. Comparative twin study on the genetic aspects of male homosexuality. *Journal of Nervous and Mental Disorders* 115:283–298.

Kelsey, J. L., and G. S. Berkowitz. 1986. Breast cancer epidemiology. *Cancer Research* 48:5615–5623.

Key, T.J.A., J. Chen, M. C. Wang, M. C. Pike, and J. Boreham. 1990. Sex hormones in women in rural China and in Britain. *British Journal of Cancer* 62:631–636.

Kimura, D. 1994. Body asymmetry and intellectual pattern. *Personality and Individual Differences* 17:53–60.

Kimura, D., and M. W. Carson. 1995. Dermatoglyphic asymmetry: Relation to sex, handedness and cognitive pattern. *Personality and Individual Differences* 19:471–478.

Kimura, M., Y. Tomita, H. Watanabe, S. Sato, and T. Abo. 1995. Androgen regulation of intra- and extra-thymic cells and its effect on sex differences in the immune system. *International Journal of Andrology* 18:127–136.

Kissebah, A. H., N. Vydelingum, R. Murray, D. J. Evans, A. J. Hartz, R. K. Kalkhoff, and P. W. Adams. 1982. Relation of body fat distribution to metabolic complications of obesity. *Journal of Clinical Endocrinology and Metabolism* 54:254–258.

Kita, E., Y. Yagyu, F. Nishikawa, A. Hamuro, D. Oku, M. Emoto, N. Katsui, and S. Kashiba. 1989. Alterations of host resistance to mouse typhoid infection by sex hormones. *Journal of Leukocyte Biology* 46:538–546.

Klein, J. M., and H. C. Nielsen. 1993. Androgen regulation of epidermal growth factor receptor binding activity during fetal rabbit lung development. *Journal of Clinical Investigation* 91:425–431.

Kleinschmidt, I. 1999. South African tuberculosis mortality data—showing the first signs of the AIDS epidemic? *South African Medical Journal* 89:269–273.

Kmietowicz, Z. 1999. Heart disease mortality declining with fewer and less-deadly attacks. *British Medical Journal* 318:1307.

Knight, B. 1991. *Forensic Pathology.* London: Edward Arnold.

Kokko, H., and J. Lindstrom. 1996. Evolution of female preference for old mates. *Proceedings of the Royal Society of London*, Series B, 263:1533–1538.

Kondo, T., J. Zakany, J. Innis, and D. Duboule. 1997. Of fingers, toes and penises. *Nature* 390:29.

Lalumiere, M. L., and M. C. Seto. 1998. What's wrong with psychopaths? *Psychiatry Rounds* 2:6.

Laverack, E. 1979. *With This Ring: 100 Years of Marriage.* London: Elm Tree Books.

Le Page, D., and M. Day. 2000. South Africa's problem with AIDS. *New Scientist* 166:14–16.

LeVay, S. 1993. *The Sexual Brain.* Cambridge, Mass.: MIT Press.

Levitt, A. J., and R. T. Joffe. 1988. Total and free testosterone in depressed men. *Acta Psychiatrica Scandinavica* 77:346–348.

Levy, E. P., A. Cohen, and F. C. Fraser. 1973. Hormone treatment during pregnancy and congenital heart defects. *Lancet* 1:611.

Lezak, M. D. 1983. *Neuropsychological Assessment.* 2d ed. New York: Oxford University Press.

Liegeois-Chauvel, C., I. Peretz, M. Babai, V. Laguitton, and P. Chauvel. 1998. Contribution of different cortical areas in the temporal lobes to music processing. *Brain* 121:1853–1867.

Links, P. S. 1980. Minor physical anomalies in childhood autism. Part II. Their relationship to maternal age. *Journal of Autism and Developmental Disorders* 10:287–292.

Links, P. S., M. Stockwell, F. Abichandani, and J. Simeon. 1980. Minor physical anomalies in childhood. Part I. Their relationship to pre- and perinatal complications. *Journal of Autism and Developmental Disorders* 10:273–285.

Logie, D. 1999. AIDS cuts life expectancy in sub-Saharan Africa by a quarter. *British Medical Journal* 319:806.

Lombard, J. 1998. Autism: A mitochondrial disorder? *Medical Hypotheses* 50:497–500.

London, W. T., and J. R. Drew. 1977. Sex differences in response to hepatitis B infection among patients receiving dialysis treatment. *Proceedings of the National Academy of Sciences* 74:2561–2563.

Lopreato, J., and M. Yu. 1988. Human fertility and fitness optimisation. *Ethology and Sociobiology* 9:269–289.

Lorber, C. A., S. B. Cassidy, and E. Engel. 1979. Is there an embryo-fetal exogenous sex steroid exposure syndrome (EFESSES)? *Fertility and Sterility* 31:21–24.

Luria, M. H., M. W. Johnson, R. Pego, C. A. Seuc, S. J. Manubens, M. R. Wieland, and R. G. Wieland. 1982. Relationship between sex hormones, myocardial infarction, and occlusive coronary disease. *Archives of Internal Medicine* 142:42–44.

MacCulloch, M. J., and J. L. Waddington. 1981. Neuroendocrine mechanisms and the etiology of male and female homosexuality. *British Journal of Psychiatry* 139:341–345.

McEwen, B. S. 1981. Neural gonadal steroid actions. *Science* 211:1303–1311.

McFadden, D. 1993. A masculinizing effect on the auditory systems of human females having male co-twins. *Proceedings of the National Academy of Sciences* 90:11900–11904.

McFadden, D. 1998. Sex differences in the auditory system. *Developmental Neuropsychology* 14:261–298.

McFadden, D., and C. A. Champlin. 2000. Comparison of auditory evoked potentials in heterosexual, homosexual and bisexual males and females. *Journal of the Association for Research in Otolaryngology* 1:89–99.

McFadden, D., and E. G. Pasanen. 1999. Spontaneous otoacoustic emissions in heterosexuals, homosexuals, and bisexuals. *Journal of the Acoustical Society of America* 105:2403–2413.

McGlone, J. 1986. The neuropsychology of sex differences in human brain organisation. *Advances in Clinical Neuropsychology* 3:1–30.

MacKlusky, N. J., and F. Naftolin. 1981. Sexual differentiation of the nervous system. *Science* 211:1294–1303.

Manning, J. T. 1985. Choosy females and correlates of male age. *Journal of Theoretical Biology* 116:349–395.

Manning, J. T. 1995. Fluctuating asymmetry and body weight in men and women: Implications for sexual selection. *Ethology and Sociobiology* 16:145–153.

Manning, J. T., R. Anderton, and S. M. Washington. 1996. Women's waists and the sex ratio of their progeny: Evolutionary aspects of the ideal female body shape. *Journal of Human Evolution* 31:41–47.

Manning, J. T., L. Barley, I. Lewis-Jones, J. Walton, R. L. Trivers, R. Thornhill, D. Singh, P. Rhode, T. Bereckzei, P. Henzi, M. Soler, and A. Sved. 2000. The 2nd to 4th digit ratio, sexual dimorphism, population differences and reproductive success: Evidence for sexually antagonistic genes. *Evolution and Human Behavior* 21:163–183.

Manning, J. T., S. Baron-Cohen, S. Wheelwright, and G. Sanders. 2001. The 2nd to 4th digit ratio and autism. *Developmental Medicine and Child Neurology* 43:160–164.

Manning, J. T., and P. Bundred. 2000. The ratio of 2nd to 4th digit length: A new predictor of disease predisposition? *Medical Hypotheses* 54:855–857.

Manning, J. T., and S. Leinster. 2001. The ratio of 2nd to 4th digit length and age at presentation of breast cancer: A link with prenatal oestrogen? *The Breast* 22:61–69.

Manning, J. T., and L. J. Pickup. 1998. Symmetry and performance in middle distance runners. *International Journal of Sports Medicine* 19:205–209.

Manning, J. T., D. Scutt, G. H. Whitehouse, S. J. Leinster, and J. M. Walton. 1996. Asymmetry and the menstrual cycle. *Ethology and Sociobiology* 17:129–143.

Manning, J. T., D. Scutt, G. H. Whitehouse, and S. J. Leinster. 1997. Breast asymmetry and phenotypic quality in women. *Evolution and Human Behavior* 18:1–13.

Manning, J. T., D. Scutt, J. Wilson, and D. I. Lewis-Jones. 1998. The ratio of 2nd to 4th digit length: A predictor of sperm numbers and levels of testosterone, LH and oestrogen. *Human Reproduction* 13:3000–3004.

Manning, J. T., and R. P. Taylor. 2001. 2nd to 4th digit ratio and male ability in sport: Implications for sexual selection in humans. *Evolution and Human Behavior* 22:61–69.

Manning, J. T., and D. J. Thompson. 1984. Muller's ratchet and favourable mutations. *Acta Biotheoretica* 33:219–225.

Manning, J. T., R. L. Trivers, D. Singh, and R. Thornhill. 1999. The mystery of female beauty. *Nature* 399:214–215.

Manning, J. T., R. L. Trivers, R. Thornhill, and D. Singh. 2000. 2nd to 4th Digit Ratio and left lateralised preference in Jamaican children. *Laterality* 5:121–132.

Markow, T. A., and K. Wandler. 1986. Fluctuating asymmetry and the genetics of liability to schizophrenia. *Psychiatric Research* 19:323–328.

Marmot, M. G., G. D. Smith, S. S. Stansfeld, C. Patel, F. North, J. Head, I. White, E. Brunner, and A. Feeney. 1991. Health inequalities among British civil servants: The Whitehall II study. *Lancet* 337:1387–1393.

Marshall, D. 2000. The heritability of 2nd to 4th digit ratio in humans. M.Sc. dissertation, University of Liverpool.

Martin, S. M., J. T. Manning, and C. F. Dowrick. 1999. Fluctuating asymmetry, relative digit length and depression in men. *Evolution and Human Behavior* 20:1–12.

Mealey, L. 1995. The sociobiology of psychopathology: An integrated evolutionary model. *Behavioral and Brain Sciences* 18:523–599.

Mendoza, S. G., A. Zerpa, H. Carrasco, O. Collomenares, A. Rangel, P. S. Gartside, and M. L. Kashyap. 1983. Estradiol, testosterone, apolipoproteins, lipoprotein cholestrol, and lipolytic enzymes in men with premature myocardial infarction and angiographically assessed coronary occlusion. *Artery* 12:1–23.

Meyer-Bahlburg, H.F.L., D. A. Boon, M. Sharma, and J. A. Edwards. 1974. Aggressiveness and testosterone measures in man. *Psychosomatic Medicine* 36:269–274.

Michaels, R. H., and K. D. Rogers. 1971. A sex difference in immunologic responsiveness. *Pediatrics* 47:120–123.

Migeon, C. J., and A. B. Wisniewski. 1998. Review—Sexual differentiation: From genes to gender. *Hormone Research* 50:245–251.

Miller, G. F. 1998. Mate choice: A cognitive perspective. *Trends in Cognitive Sciences* 2:161–201.

Miller, G. F. 2000. Evolution of human music through sexual selection. In *The Origins of Music*, ed. N. L. Wallin, B. Merker, and S. Brown. Cambridge, Mass.: MIT Press.

Miller, G. F., and P. M. Todd. 1995. The role of mate choice in biocomputation: Sexual selection as a process of search, optimization and diversification. In

Evolution and Biocomputation: Computational Models of Evolution, ed. W. Banzaff and F. Eeckman. Berlin: Springer-Verlag, 27–38.

Minshew, N. J., G. Goldstein, S. M. Dombrowski, K. Panchalingam, and J. W. Pettegrew. 1993. A preliminary 31PMSR study of autism: Evidence for under-synthesis and increased degredation of brain membranes. *Biological Psychiatry* 33:762–773.

Mittwoch, U., and S. Mahadevaiah. 1980. Additional growth: A link between mammalian testes, avian ovaries, gonadal asymmetry in hermaphrodites and the expression of H-Y antigen. *Growth* 44:287–300.

Møller, A. P., M. Soler, and R. Thornhill. 1995. Breast asymmetry, sexual selection and human reproductive success. *Ethology and Sociobiology* 16:207–219.

Money, J., M. Schwartz, and V. C. Lewis. 1984. Adult eroto sexual status and fetal hormonal masculinization: 46,XX congenital virilizing adrenal hypoplasia and 46,XY androgen insensitivity syndrome compared. *Psychoneuroendocrinology* 9:405–411.

Morishima, A., M. M. Grumbach, E. R. Simpson, C. Fisher, and K. Qin. 1995. Aromatase deficiency in male and female siblings caused by a novel mutation and the physiological role of estrogens. *Journal of Clinical Endocrinolgy and Metabolism* 80:3689–3698.

Mortlock, D. P., and J. W. Innis. 1997. Mutation of *Hoxa13* in hand-foot-genital syndrome. *Nature Genetics* 15:179–180.

Mortlock, D. P., J. W. Innis, and L. C. Post. 1996. The molecular basis of hypodactyly (Hd), a deletion in *Hoxa13* leads to arrest of digital arch formation. *Nature Genetics* 13:284–289.

Mota, E. A., C. W. Todd, J. H. Maguire, D. Portugal, O. O. Santana, R. R. Filho, and I. A. Sherlock. 1984. Megaesophagus and seroreactivity to *Trypanosoma cruzi* in a rural community in northeast Brazil. *American Journal of Tropical Medicine and Hygeine* 33:820–826.

Mueller, U., and A. Mazur. 1997. Facial dominance in Homo sapiens as honest signaling of male quality. *Behavioral Ecology* 5:569–579.

Neligan, G. A., T. Kolvin, D. M. Scott, and R. F. Garside. 1976. Born too soon or born too small. *Clinics in Developmental Medicine* 61. London: Spastics International Medical Publications.

Nora, J. J., A. H. Nora, A. G. Perinchief, J. W. Ingram, A. K. Fountain, and M. J. Peterson. 1976. Congenital abnormalities and first-trimester exposure to progestogen/oestrogen. *Lancet* 1:313–314.

Norton, S. J. 1992. The effects of being a newborn on otoacoustic emissions. *Journal of the Acoustical Society of America* (Supplement 1) 91:2409.

Ogloff, J.R.P., and S. Wong. 1990. Electrodermal and cardiovascular evidence of coping response in psychopaths. *Criminal Justice and Behavior* 17:231–245.

Oliveira, J.S.M., J. A. Mello de Oliveira, U. Frederiques, and E. C. Lima Filho. 1981. Apical aneurism of Chagas' heart disease. *British Heart Journal* 46:432–437.

Olweus, D., A. Mattson, D. Scalling, and H. Low. 1980. Testosterone, aggression, physical and personality dimensions in normal adolescent males. *Psychosomatic Medicine* 42:253–269.

Patrick, C. J. 1994. Emotion and psychopathy: Startling new insights. *Psychophysiology* 31:319–330.

Patrick, C. J., and K. A. Zempolich. 1998. Emotion and aggression in the psychopathic personality. *Aggression and Violent Behavior* 3:303–338.

Patty, D. W., J. Furesz, and D. W. Boucher. 1976. Measles antibodies as related to HLA types in multiple sclerosis. *Neurology* 26:651–655.

Pawlowski, B., R.I.M. Dunbar, and A. Lipowicz. 2000. Tall men have more reproductive success. *Nature* 403:156.

Peichel, C. L., B. Prabhakaran, and T. F. Vogt. 1997. The mouse *Ulnaless* mutation deregulates posterior *Hoxd* gene expression and alters appendicular patterning. *Development* 24:3481–3492.

Penrose, L. S. 1967. Finger-print pattern and the sex chromosomes. *Lancet* 1:298–300.

Peretz, I. 1990. Processing of local and global musical information by unilateral brain-damaged patients. *Brain* 113:1185–1205.

Peters, M., K. Mackenzie, and P. Bryden. 2002. Finger length patterns in humans. *American Journal of Physical Anthropology*.

Pfitzner, W. 1892. Beitrage zur kentniss des menschlichen exstremitatenskelets. V. Anthropologische Beziehungen der Hand- und Fussmaasse. *Morphologische Arbeiten* 1:1–120.

Phelps, V. R. 1952. Relative index finger length as a sex-influenced trait in man. *American Journal of Human Genetics* 4:72–89.

Phillips, G. B., T. Y. Jing, and J. H. Laragh, 1997. Serum sex hormone levels in postmenopausal women with hypertension. *Journal of Human Hypertension* 11:523–526.

Phillips, G. B., B. H. Pinkernell, and T. Y. Jing. 1994. The association of hypotestosteronemia with coronary artery disease in men. *Arteriosclerosis and Thrombosis* 14:701–706.

Pilgrim, C., and J. Reisert. 1992. Differences between male and female brains: Developmental mechanisms and implications. *Hormonal and Metabolic Research* 24:353–359.

Pillard, R. C., and J. D. Weinrich. 1987. The periodic table model of the gender transpositions, I: A theory based on masculinisation and defeminisation of the brain. *Journal of Sexual Research* 23:425–454.

Raine, A. 1993. *The Psychopathology of Crime.* San Diego, Calif.: Academic Press.

Ramesh, A., and J. S. Murty. 1977. Variation and inheritance of relative length of index finger in man. *Annals of Human Biology* 4:479–484.

Reay-Young, P. S., and M. Chir. 1974. Clinical experience of Burkitt's lymphoma in Papua, New Guinea. *Australian Radiology* 18:387–392.

Reber, A. S. 1985. *The Penguin Dictionary of Psychology.* London: Penguin Books.

Rhodes, K., R. L. Markham, P. M. Maxwell, and M. E. Monks Jones. 1969. Immunoglobulins and the X-chromosome. *British Medical Journal* iii:439–441.

Rice, T., D. L. Sprecher, I. B. Borecki, L. E. Mitchell, P. M. Laskarzewski, and D. C. Rao. 1993. Cincinnati myocardial infarction and hormone family study: Family resemblance for testosterone in random and myocardial infarction families. *American Journal of Medical Genetics* 47:542–549.

Rice, W. R. 1996a. Evolution of the Y sex chromosome in animals. *BioScience* 46:331–343.

Rice, W. R. 1996b. Sexually antagonistic male adaptation triggered by experimental arrest of female evolution. *Nature* 381:232–234.

Rice, W. R., and B. Holland. 1997. The enemies within: Intergenomic conflict, interlocus contest evolution (ICE), and the intraspecific Red Queen. *Behavioral Ecology and Sociobiology* 41:1–10.

Robertson, D.H.H. 1963. Human trypanosomiasis in south-east Uganda. *Bulletin of the World Health Organization* 28:627–643.

Robinson, S. J., and J. T. Manning. 2000. The ratio of 2nd to 4th digit length and male homosexuality. *Evolution and Human Behavior* 21:333–345.

Rodier, P. M., S. E. Bryson, and J. P. Welch. 1997. Minor malformations and physical measurements in autism: Data from Nova Scotia. *Teratology* 55:319–325.

Romer, A. S. 1966. *Vertebrate Paleontology*. Chicago: University of Chicago Press.

Rosamond, W. D., L. E. Chambless, A. R. Folsom, L. S. Cooper, D. E. Conwill, L. Clegg, C. H. Wang, and G. Heiss. 1998. Trends in the incidence of myocardial infarction and in mortality due to coronary heart disease. *New England Journal of Medicine* 339:861–867.

Rosano, G.M.C. 2000. Androgens and coronary artery disease: A sex-specific effect of sex hormones? *European Heart Journal* 21:868–871.

Ross, R., L. Bernstein, H. R. Judd, R. Hanisch, M. Pike, and B. Henderson. 1986. Serum testosterone levels in healthy young black and white men. *Journal of the National Cancer Institute* 76:45–48.

Rowe, D. S., I. A. McGregor, S. J. Smith, P. Hall, and K. Williams. 1968. Plasma immunoglobulin concentrations in a West African (Gambian) community and in a healthy group of British adults. *Clinical and Experimental Immunology* 3:63–79.

Ruse, M. 1981. Are there gay genes? Sociobiology and homosexuality. *Journal of Homosexuality* 6:5–34.

Rutter, M. 1978. Diagnosis and definition. In *Autism: A Reappraisal of Concepts and Treatment*, ed. M. Rutter and E. Schopler. New York: Plenum Press.

Sadalla, E. K., D. T. Kenrick, and B. Vershure. 1987. Dominance and heterosexual attraction. *Journal of Personality and Social Psychology* 52:730–738.

Sadler, T. W. 1985. *Langman's Medical Embryology*. 5th ed. Baltimore: Williams and Wilkins, 1985.

Sanders, G., and L. Ross-Field. 1986. Sexual orientation and visuo-spatial ability. *Brain and Cognition* 5:280–290.

Sanders, G., and D. Wenmoth. 1998. Verbal and music dichotic listening tasks reveal variations in functional cerebral asymmetry across the menstrual cycle that are phase- and task- dependent. *Neuropsychologia* 36:869–874.

Sanderson, M., M. A. Williams, K. E. Malone, J. L. Stanford, I. Emanuel, and E. White. 1996. Perinatal factors and risk of breast cancer. *Epidemiology* 7:34–37.

Schlegel, W. S. 1975. Parameter beckenskellet. *Sexualmedizin* 4:228–232.

Schultz, A. H. 1924. Growth studies on primates bearing upon man's evolution. *American Journal of Physical Anthropology* 7:149–164.

Schwabl, H. 1996. Environment modifies the testosterone levels of a female bird and its eggs. *Journal of Experimental Zoology* 276:157–163.

Scott, M. P. 1997. *Hox* genes, arms and the man. *Nature Genetics* 15:117–118.

Scutt, D., and J. T. Manning. 1996. Symmetry and ovulation in women. *Human Reproduction* 11:2477–2480.

Scutt, D., J. T. Manning, G. H. Whitehouse, S. J. Leinster, and C. P. Massey. 1997. The relationship between breast asymmetry, breast size and the occurrence of breast cancer. *British Journal of Radiology* 70:1017–1021.

Sewdarsen, M., I. Jailal, S. Vythilingum, and R. K. Desai. 1986. Sex hormone levels in young Indian patients with myocardial infarction. *Arteriosclerosis* 6:418–421.

Sewdarsen, M., S. Vylithingum, I. Jailal, R. K. Desai, and P. Becker. 1990. Abnormalities in sex hormones are a risk factor for premature manifestation of coronary artery disease in South African Indian men. *Athersclerosis* 83:111–117.

Shubin, N. H., and P. Alberch. 1986. A morphogenetic approach to the origin and basic organisation of the tetrapod limb. *Evolutionary Biology* 20:319–387.

Simpson, E. R., M. S. Mahendroo, G. D. Means, M. W. Kilgore, M. M. Hinshelwood, S. Graham-Lorence, B. Amarneh, Y. Ito, C. R. Fisher, M. D. Michael, C. R. Mendelson, and S. E. Bulun. 1994. Aromatase cyrochrome P450, the enzyme responsible for estrogen biosynthesis. *Endocrinology Review* 15:342–355.

Singh, D. 1993. Adaptive significance of female physical attractiveness: Role of waist-to-hip ratio. *Journal of Personality and Social Psychology* 65:293–307.

Singh, D., and R. K. Young. 1995. Body weight, waist-to-hip ratio, breasts and hips: Role in judgements of female attractiveness and desirability for relationships. *Ethology and Sociobiology* 16:483–507.

Singh, D., and R. J. Zambarano. 1997. Offspring sex ratio in women with android body fat distribution. *Human Biology* 69:545–556.

Sluming, V. A., and J. T. Manning. 2000. Second to fourth digit ratio in elite musicians: Evidence for musical ability as an honest signal of male fitness. *Evolution and Human Behavior* 21:1–9.

Smith, G.C.S., M.F.S. Smith, M. B. McNay, and J.E.E. Fleming. 1998. First trimester growth and the risk of low birth weight. *New England Journal of Medicine* 339:1817–1822.

Sorell, W. 1968. *The Story of the Human Hand*. London: Weidenfeld and Nicholson.

Spencer, M. J., J. D. Chery, K. R. Powell, M. R. Mickey, P. I. Terasaki, S. M. Mary, and C. V. Sumaya. 1977. Antibody responses following rubella immunization analyzed by HLA and ABO types. *Immunogenetics* 4:365–372.

Staines, N. A., J. Brostoff, and K. James. 1992. *Introducing Immunology*. 2d ed. London: Mosby.

Steer, R. A., A. T. Beck, and B. Garrison. 1985. Applications of the Beck Depression Inventory. In *Assessment of Depression*, ed. N. Sartorius and T. A. Banta. New York: Springer-Verlag.

Steiger, A., F. Holsboer, and O. Benkert. 1993. Studies of nocturnal penile tumescence and sleep encephalogram in patients with major depression and normal controls. *Acta Psychiatrica Scandinavica* 87:358–363.

Stevenson, C. J., P. Blackburn, and P.O.D. Pharaoh. 1999. Longitudinal study of behaviour disorders in low birth weight infants. *Archives of Disease in Childhood and Fetal Neonatology* 81:5–9.

Stoller, R. J., and G. H. Herdt. 1985. Theories of origins of male homosexuality: A cross-cultural look. *Archives of General Psychiatry* 42:399–404.

Suominen, J., and M. Vierula. 1993. Semen quality of Finnish men. *British Medical Journal* 306:1579.

Swartz, C. M., and M. A. Young. 1987. Low serum testosterone and myocardial infarction in geriatric male patients. *Journal of American Geriatrics Society* 35:39–44.

Tanner, J. M. 1990. *Foetus into Man: Physical Growth from Conception to Maturity.* Cambridge, Mass.: Harvard University Press.

Thornhill, R., and S. W. Gangestad. 1994. Fluctuating asymmetry and human sexual behavior. *Psychological Science* 5:297–302.

Thornhill, R., S. W. Gangestad, and D. Comer. 1995. Human female orgasm and mate fluctuating asymmetry. *Animal Behavior* 50:1601–1615.

Townsend, P., P. Phillimore, and A. Beatie. 1988. *Health and Deprivation: Inequality in the North.* London: Croom Helm.

Trichopoulos, D. 1990. Does breast cancer originate in utero? *Lancet* 335:939–940.

Trichopoulos, D., S. Yen, J. Brown, P. Cole, and B. MacMahon. 1984. The effect of westernization on urine estrogens, frequency of ovulation and breast cancer risk. *Cancer* 53:187–192.

Trivers, R. L., J. T. Manning, R. Thornhill, D. Singh, and M. McGuire. 1999. Jamaican Symmetry Project: Long-term study of fluctuating asymmetry in rural Jamaican children. *Human Biology* 71:419–432.

Van den Hoogen, P.C.W., E.J.M. Feskens, N.J.D. Nagelkerke, A. A. Menotti, A. Nissinen, and D. Kromhout. 2000. The relation between blood pressure and mortality due to coronary heart disease among men in different parts of the world. *New England Journal of Medicine* 342:1–8.

Varley, R. 1995. Lexical semantic deficits following right hemisphere damage: Evidence from verbal fluency tasks. *European Journal of Disorders of Communication* 30:362–371.

Veatch, E. P. 1946. Human trypanosomiasis and tsetse flies in Liberia. *American Journal of Tropical Medicine* 26:supplement, 5–52.

Videbech, P. 1997. MRI findings in patients with affective disorder: A meta-analysis. *Acta Psychiatrica Scandinavica* 96:157–168.

Vierula, M., M. Niemi, M. Keiski, M. Saaranen, S. Saarikoski, and J. Souminen. 1996. High and unchanged sperm counts of Finnish men. *International Journal of Andrology* 19:11–17.

Vogel, W., F. L. Klaiber, and D. M. Broverman. 1978. Roles of the gonadal steroid hormones in psychiatric depression in men and women. *Progress in Neuropsychopharmacology* 2:487–503.

Voyer, D. 1996. On the magnitude of laterality effects and sex differences in functional brain lateralities. *Laterality* 1:51–83.

Walker, H. A. 1976. Dermatoglyphic patterns in infantile autism. In M. Coleman, ed., *The Autistic Syndromes,* 117–134. Amsterdam: North-Holland.

Waynforth, D. 1998. Fluctuating asymmetry and human male life-history traits in rural Belize. *Proceedings of the Royal Society of London,* B Series, 265:1497–1501.

Webb, C. M., D. L. Adamson, D. de Zeigler, and P. Collins. 1999. Effects of testosterone on coronary vasomotor regulation in men with coronary heart disease. *Circulation* 100:1690–1696.

Wei, M., S. P. Gaskill, S. M. Haffner, and M. P. Stern. 1997. Waist circumference as the best predictor of non–insulin-dependent diabetes melitus (NIDDM) compared to body mass index, waist:hip ratio and other anthropometric measurements in Mexican Americans: A seven-year prospective study. *Obesity Research* 5:16–23.

Wei, M., S. P. Gaskill, S. M. Haffner, and M. P. Stern. 1998. Effects of diabetes and level of glycemia on all-cause cardiovascular mortality. *Diabetes Care* 21:1167–1172.

Weinrich, J. D. 1987. A new sociobiological theory of homosexuality applicable to societies with universal marriage. *Ethology and Sociobiology* 8:37–47.

Wexler, L. A. 1999. Studies of acute coronary syndromes in women: Lessons for everyone. *New England Journal of Medicine* 341:275–276.

Williamson, S., T. J. Harpur, and R. D. Hare. 1991. Abnormal processing of affective words by psychopaths. *Journal of Psychophysiological Research* 28:260–273.

Wilson, J. M., and J. T. Manning. 1996. Fluctuating asymmetry and age in children: Evolutionary implications for the control of developmental stability. *Journal of Human Evolution* 30:529–537.

Wing, L. 1981. Asperger Syndrome: A clinical account. *Psychological Medicine* 11:115–130.

Williams, T. J., M. E. Pepitone, S. E. Christensen, B. M. Cooke, A. D. Huberman, N. J. Breedlove, T. J. Breedlove, C. L. Jordan, and S. M. Breedlove. 2000. Finger length patterns indicate an influence of fetal androgens on human sexual orientation. *Nature* 404:455.

Williamson, S., T. J. Harpur, and R. D. Hare. 1987. Abnormal processing of affective words by psychopaths. *Journal of Psychophysiological Research* 28:260–273.

Wilson, G. D. 1983. Finger length as an index of assertiveness in women. *Personality and Individual Differences* 4:111–112.

Winkler, E. M., and K. Christiansen. 1993. Sex hormone levels and body hair growth in !Kung San and Kavango men from Namibia. *American Journal of Physical Anthropology* 92:155–164.

Wood-Jones, F. 1941. *The Principles of Anatomy as Seen in the Hand.* 2d ed. Baltimore: Williams and Wilkins.

World Health Organization. 1987. *Expert Committee on Onchocerciasis.* Geneva: World Health Organization, Technical Report series, no. 725.

World Health Organization, MONICA Project. 1988. Geographical variation in the major risk factors of coronary heart disease in men and women aged 35–64 years. *World Health Statistics Quarterly* 41:115–140.

Wright, S. P. 1992. Adjusted P-values for simultaneous inference. *Biometrics* 48:1005–1013.

Wu, F. 1983. Endocrinology of male infertility and fertility. In *Male Infertility*, ed. T. B. Hargreave. Berlin: Springer-Verlag, 87–111.

Wynder, E. L., I. J. Bross, and T. Hirayama. 1960. A study of the epidemiology of cancer of the breast. *Cancer* 130:559–601.

Yu, D. W., and G. H. Sheppard. 1998. Is beauty in the eye of the beholder? *Nature* 396:321–322.

Yue, P., K. Chatterjee, C. Beale, A. Poole-Wilson, and P. Collins. 1995. Testosterone relaxes rabbit coronary arteries and aorta. *Circulation* 91:1154–1160.

Zahavi, A. 1975. Mate selection: A selection for a handicap. *Journal of Theoretical Biology* 53:205–214.

Zahavi, A. 1977. The cost of honesty (further remarks on the handicap principle). *Journal of Theoretical Biology* 67:603–605.

Zar, J. 1994. *Biostatistical Analysis*. Englewood Cliffs, N.J.: Prentice-Hall.

Zicker, F., P. G. Smith, J. C. Almeida Netto, R. M. Oliveira, and E.M.S. Zicker. 1990. Physical activity, opportunity for reinfection, and sibling history of heart disease as risk factors for Chagas' cardiopathy. *American Journal of Tropical Medicine and Hygiene* 43:498–505.

Zimmer, C. 1998. *At the Water's Edge*. London: Touchstone.

Zmuda, J. M., J. A. Cauley, A. Kriska, N. W. Glynn, J. P. Gutai, and L. H. Kuller. 1997. Longitudinal relation between endogenous testosterone and cardiovascular disease risk factors in middle-aged men: A 13-year follow up of former Multiple Risk Factor Intervention Trial participants. *American Journal of Epidemiology* 146:609–617.

Index

Acanthostega, 17
Adams, M. R., 83
adrenal glands, 31
age: attractiveness and, 48, 49; breast cancer and, 89, 91; gestational, 80; musical ability and, 115, 120; myocardial infarction and, 85–89, 88*tab;* sexual orientation and, 104–105; status and, 43; testosterone and, 25
aggression, xiv, 41, 142; cortisol and, 41; pelvic structure and, 42; status and, 41, 142; testosterone and, 41, 44; 2D:4D and, 44–47
AIDS. *See* HIV/AIDS
Ainbender, E., 96
Aksut, S. V., 84
Alexandersen, P., 83
allergies, 94
Alouatta palliata, 18
Anderson, T. J., 90
androgen: adrenal, 101; birth weight and, 77–78; brain organization and, 62, 63; insensitivity to, 102; prenatal, 102; receptors for, 63; reproductive system development and, 54; sensitivity to, 30
androgenization, 30, 32
Archer, J., 41, 44, 45
aromatase, 25, 63, 90, 110
Arrieta, I., 69
Asperger Syndrome, 68
assertiveness, xiv; in females, 41–42; 2D:4D and, 41–42
asthma, 93
asymmetry: breast, xiii, 22, 90; cognitive patterns and, 22; fluctuating, 49, 124; nervous system, 63; of ridge counts, 35; testicular, 22
atherosclerosis, 83
athletic ability, 126–140
atrial septal defect, 85
attractiveness: age and, 48, 49;

dominance behavior and, 47; fluctuating asymmetry and, 49; height and, 48; predictors of, 49*tab;* 2D:4D and, 47–51; weight and, 48
autism, xv, 68–71; biological theory of, 69; causes of, 69; "extreme male brain theory" of, 69; hemisphere enhancements in, 68; heritability of, 68, 70, 71*fig;* incidence of, 68; "islets" of ability in, 68; minor physical anomalies in, 69; musical ability and, 116; psychogenic theory of, 69; testosterone and, 62, 68; in twins, 69; 2D:4D and, 12, 68–71; waist:hip ratio and, 71
autoimmunity, 94

Bailey, M. J., 68, 69, 95, 100, 113
Baker, F., xiii, 7
baldness, 11
Banks, T., 44
Bardin, C. W., 62, 63
Barker, D.J.B., 76, 78, 82, 85, 144
Baron-Cohen, S., 68, 69, 70, 116
Barrett-Connor, E., 84
Beck Depression Inventory, 72, 73, 73*fig,* 74*tab*
Bell, A. P., 37, 100, 101, 104, 113
Bettelheim, B., 69
Biedle-Bardet syndrome, 69
birth order, 109–113
birth weight, 76, 77–82; androgens and, 77–78; developmental patterns and, 77–78; as disease correlate, 76, 78; estrogen and, 78, 90; heart disease and, 82; intelligence and, 81–82; normal, 81; testosterone and, 78; 2D:4D and, 79–82
bisexuality, 101
Bjorntorp, P., 31
Blanchard, R., 109, 110
blood pressure, 82, 85
Bogaert, A. F., 102, 109

172   INDEX

status (*continued*)
   socioeconomic, 43; in sports, 126;
   testosterone and, 43; 2D:4D and,
   43, 142; valued by women, 47
Steer, R. A., 73
Steiger, A., 72
Stevenson, C. J., 82
Stoller, R. J., 100
stress, prenatal, 10
suicide, 72
supraorbital ridges, 5, 20
Swartz, C. M., 84
Sweden: mental rotation studies in, 131,
   132
syndactyly, 6

tamoxifen, 90
Tanner, J. M., 6, 9, 21, 22, 27, 76
Tcherepnin, Alexander, 121
testes, development of, 6, 24
testosterone: age and, 25; aggression
   and, 41, 44; allergies and, 94;
   autism and, 68; birth weight and,
   78; brain and, 62–63; depression
   and, 72; diabetes and, 93; dyslexia
   and, 43; effects of, xiii; estradiol
   and, 62, 63; in females, 31–35, 49;
   fertility and, 49; fetal, xiii; free, 32;
   genes for production of, 31;
   handedness and, 37, 63, 78; heart
   disease and, 83–85; height and, 25;
   hirsute digits and, 30–31; homosexuality and, 94; immune system
   and, 94; luteinizing hormone and,
   38, 39; masculinization and, 101;
   myocardial infarction and, 83–84;
   negative effects of, 62; nervous
   system damage and, 62; nervous
   system development and, 78; non-
   SHBG-bound, 35; obesity and, 25;
   population differences and, 35–37;
   prenatal, 18, 63, 69, 72, 76, 94, 95,
   100, 145; production of, 24, 30;
   sources of, 31; status and, 43; 2D:4D
   and, xiii, xiv, 24–40; in utero, 65; as
   vasodilator, 84; verbal ability and,
   43; weight and, 25, 26
Thornhill, R., 124
"throwing ape," 16

thumbs, fingerization of, 39
thymus gland, 78
thyroid gland, 78
Townsend, P., 43
Townsend Deprivation Score, 44
Trichopoulos, D., 90
triglycerides, 84
Trivers, R. L., 6
Trypanosoma cruzi, 97
trypanosomiasis, 77
tuberculosis, 94
Tulerpeton, 17
2D:3D ratio, 12; sexual dimorphism and,
   30–31
2D:4D ratio: academic ability and, 143–
   144; aggression and, 44–47;
   androgenization and, 30–31;
   assertiveness and, 41–42; assessing
   competitiveness and, 41; assortative
   pairing and, 50, 50*fig*; athletic
   ability and, 126–140; attractiveness
   and, 47–51; autism and, xv, 12, 68–
   71; birth weight and, 9, 10, 79–82;
   breast cancer and, 89–91, 92*fig*;
   central nervous system and, 143–
   144; changes in, 14, 15*fig*; courtship
   and, 16; cross-cultural tests of
   mental rotation and, 131–132;
   depression and, xv, 44, 71–74;
   deprivation and, 43, 44*fig*; derma-
   tolglyphic ridges and, 9, 10, 11*fig*;
   determining factors, 24–40; diabetes
   and, 91–93; disease and, xiv, 144–
   145; endometrial cancer and, 93;
   establishment of, 13–14; estrogen
   and, xiv, 24–40; ethnic differences,
   19, 20, 21, 35–37; father-child
   relationships, 22; in females, xiii, 7,
   8*fig*; fertility and, xiv, 53, 55–62,
   142–143; fixation prenatally, 25;
   football and, 132–140; forearm and,
   9; future research, 141–146;
   handedness and, xv, 21–22, 27–30,
   63–65; heart disease and, xv, 82;
   height and, 7; heritability of, 10, 12;
   hirsute digits and, 30–31; HIV/AIDS
   and, 77, 93–95; homosexuality and,
   xv, 103–109; in human populations,
   18–21; immune system and, 93–95;

About the Author

John Manning graduated with a bachelor's degree in zoology from London University and with a master's degree in evolutionary biology and a doctorate in animal behavior from the University of Liverpool. He is a reader in the School of Biological Sciences at the University of Liverpool, and he has published extensively in the area of the evolution of sex, sexual selection in crustacea, sex differences in cradling behavior, and developmental stability and sexual selection in humans. In 1998 he suggested that the 2nd to 4th digit ratio was a marker for prenatal exposure to testosterone and estrogen and began an extensive series of investigations into the ratio.